"An important and hopeful contribution clinicians can facilitate a woman's struggle to grow through the process of birthing and parenting. The psychological and corporeal challenges and possibilities make this required as well as illuminating reading."

Susie Orbach, PhD, *author of* Fat is a Feminist Issue *and* Bodies

"In this brilliantly conceived and passionate book, Vissing brings a long overdue integration of analytic relational thinking with somatic psychology to bear on women's perinatal difficulties, offering a trenchant analysis of the barriers to the recognition of maternal suffering along with an inspiring account of essential clinical strategies for treatment. Truly vital reading for anyone concerned with the psychological and biosocial world of mothers and infants."

Jessica Benjamin, PhD, *author of* The Bonds of Love *and* Beyond Doer and Done To

"*Somatic Maternal Healing* expertly presents a trauma-informed, research-based framework to better understand the transition to motherhood within the context of profound change, adaptation, and transformation. All therapists working in the field of maternal mental health should have access to these compelling and essential clinical interpretations and interventions."

Karen Kleiman, LCSW, *author of* The Art of Holding in Therapy

Somatic Maternal Healing

Somatic Maternal Healing introduces a cutting-edge understanding of the body into the growing field of perinatal mental health. Chapters lay out a complete trauma treatment model for maternal mental health, integrating psychodynamic and somatic clinical techniques within a systemic perspective. The book applies a biopsychosocial conceptualization of mental health in the perinatal period with a special emphasis on trauma and somatic trauma treatment.

Somatic Maternal Healing is for anyone working clinically with mothers and new families, specifically therapists, clinical social workers, psychologists, psychoanalysts, psychiatrists, researchers, academics, clinical educators, and graduate students and trainees within these fields.

Helena Vissing, PsyD, SEP, PMH-C, is a licensed psychologist and Somatic Experiencing® practitioner based in Northern California. She is certified in perinatal mental health and specializes in trauma treatment and psychodynamic psychotherapy.

Somatic Maternal Healing

Psychodynamic and Somatic Trauma Treatment for Perinatal Mental Health

By Helena Vissing

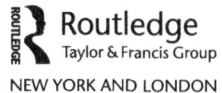
Routledge
Taylor & Francis Group
NEW YORK AND LONDON

Cover image: © Getty Images

First published 2024
by Routledge
605 Third Avenue, New York, NY 10158

and by Routledge
4 Park Square, Milton Park, Abingdon, Oxon, OX14 4RN

Routledge is an imprint of the Taylor & Francis Group, an informa business

© 2024 Helena Vissing

The right of Helena Vissing to be identified as author of this work has been asserted in accordance with sections 77 and 78 of the Copyright, Designs and Patents Act 1988.

All rights reserved. No part of this book may be reprinted or reproduced or utilised in any form or by any electronic, mechanical, or other means, now known or hereafter invented, including photocopying and recording, or in any information storage or retrieval system, without permission in writing from the publishers.

Trademark notice: Product or corporate names may be trademarks or registered trademarks, and are used only for identification and explanation without intent to infringe.

Library of Congress Cataloging-in-Publication Data
Names: Vissing, Helena, author.
Title: Somatic maternal healing : psychodynamic and somatic trauma treatment for perinatal mental health / by Helena Vissing.
Description: New York, NY : Routledge, 2024. | Includes bibliographical references and index. |
Identifiers: LCCN 2023016126 (print) | LCCN 2023016127 (ebook) | ISBN 9781032315225 (hardback) | ISBN 9781032315249 (paperback) | ISBN 9781003310914 (ebook)
Subjects: LCSH: Mothers--Psychology. | Mothers--Mental health. | Motherhood--Psychological aspects.
Classification: LCC HQ759 .V57 2023 (print) | LCC HQ759 (ebook) | DDC 306.874/3--dc23/eng/20230428
LC record available at https://lccn.loc.gov/2023016126
LC ebook record available at https://lccn.loc.gov/2023016127

ISBN: 978-1-032-31522-5 (hbk)
ISBN: 978-1-032-31524-9 (pbk)
ISBN: 978-1-003-31091-4 (ebk)

DOI: 10.4324/9781003310914

Typeset in Palatino
by MPS Limited, Dehradun

to Zoë, for letting me listen
and
to Ash and Luna,
for all our shared femaleness
in our perinatal transitions

Contents

List of Figures and Tables xv
Acknowledgments xvi
List of Abbreviations xix

Introduction: Why We Need Maternal Healing that Includes Self, Body, and Society 1
Outline of the Book 13

Part I **Introduction to Part I: Overview of Trauma in the Perinatal Period** 19
Defining Traumatic Stress and Trauma 19
Trauma and the Perinatal Period 23
Types of Perinatal Trauma 26
    Childhood Maltreatment 26
    Preterm Delivery 27
    Traumatic Childbirth and Iatrogenic Effects of Obstetric Care 27
    Pregnancy and Infant Loss and Stillbirth 29
    Discrimination and Health Inequity 30
    Sexual Abuse 31
    Intimate Partner Violence (IPV) 32
    Disasters and Pandemic Stress 33
Trauma Symptoms from a Perinatal Perspective 33
    Delayed Onset 35
    Sleep Disturbances 36
    Flashbacks and Intrusive Thoughts 38
    Avoidance and Dissociation 39
    Negative Mood or Cognitions 41
    Hyperarousal and Reactivity 42
    Anger, Rage, and Irritability 43

Suicidality 44
A Biopsychosocial Approach to Trauma-Informed
Perinatal Care 45

**1 The Question of Embodied Maternal
Subjectivity: How Feminist Psychoanalysis
Informs Clinical Work with Mothers** 60
From Developmental Tasks of Maternal Identity
Formation to Embodied Relational Subjectivity 60
The Maternal Subjectivity Problem 62
The Maternal Body Problem and Trauma 67
Mothering from a Traumatized Body Self 69
It All Comes Back to the (Maternal) Body: How
Relational Psychoanalysis Brings the Body into
Perinatal Clinical Work 71

**2 Understanding Trauma in Light of the
Biological Changes of Motherhood** 79
"Mommy Brain" Revisited: Trauma-Informed
Understanding of the Biological Adaptations
of the Maternal Transition 79
How Trauma is Nuancing Our Understanding
of Oxytocin 80
The Overlap Between Perinatal Changes, PMADs,
and Trauma Biology: HPA Axis Dysregulation
and Inflammation 81
Traumatic Childbirth 83
Connecting the Dots: The Causal Loops of
Perinatal Trauma and Reproductive Biology 84
Implications for Trauma-Responsive Maternal
Mental Health: Fighting Inflammation with
Stress-Reduction and Adopting a Plasticity
Perspective 85

3 **Resisting Patriarchal Motherhood: From Maternal Bodylessness to Maternal Bodyfulness** 92
The Institution of Motherhood and the Emergence of Matricentric Feminism 92
Intensive Mothering and the Dictates of Patriarchal Motherhood 94
Matricentric Feminism and Feminist Psychoanalysis 97
How Intensive Mothering Ideology Affects Maternal Mental Health 98
Feminist and Empowered Mothering 101
Somatic Consequences of Patriarchal Motherhood: Maternal Bodylessness 104
Body Identity and Bodyfulness 106
Maternal Bodyfulness as Empowered Mothering 108
Matricentric Feminist Mothering, Somatic Psychology, and Perinatal Trauma-Healing 111

4 **Rationale and Principles of Somatic Maternal Healing** 115
From Top-Down to Bottom-Up: Neuroscientific Advances in Traumatology 115
The Bottom-Up Approach to Trauma Treatment: The Scientific Background for Somatic Psychotherapy 118
The Heightened Risks for Trauma in the Perinatal Period 122
From Vulnerability to Opportunity 126
The Rationale for Somatic Interventions in Maternal Mental Health 127
Integrating Psychodynamic Psychotherapy and Somatic Psychotherapy 130

Part II Introduction to Part II: Principles, Treatment Goals, and Key Clinical Skills of Maternal Somatic Healing................................. 139
  Integrating Feminist Psychoanalysis, Matricentric Feminism, and Somatic Psychology............... 139
  The Principles of Somatic Maternal Healing....... 140
  Psychological 140
  Biological..................................... 141
  Social 141
  Treatment Goals and Strategy: Maternal Bodyfulness 142
  Key Clinical Skills................................ 144

5 Working Somatically in the Perinatal Transferential Field 147
  Attunement and Empathy in the Perinatal Context... 147
  Resonance and the New Mother.................. 150
  How Trauma Impacts Perinatal Coregulation...... 152
  Coregulation and Shame........................ 154
  Key Clinical Skill of Somatic Attunement and Resonance 155
  Nervous System Tracking........................ 157
  Sitting with the Dysregulation of the Perinatal Period... 160
  Somatic Receptivity 163
  How Trauma Interferes with Somatic Receptivity 164
  Somatic Countertransference 167
  Somatic Attunement and Resonance in Perinatal Telehealth 170
  Clinician Self-Reflection........................... 172

6 Maternal Bodyfulness: Working with Perinatal Sensory Awareness and Vocabulary 176
  Emotion Regulation and Sensory Awareness in the Perinatal Period.......................... 176

Maternal Sense of Self, Sensory Awareness,
and Pleasure 182
The Impact of Perinatal Trauma on Sensory
Awareness and the Therapeutic Relationship 184
Introducing Sensory Awareness Skills to
Perinatal Clients 188
Somatic Self-Regulation Skills 189
Sensory Vocabulary and Maternal Body
Narrative 191
Maternal Bodyfulness Themes in Trauma Healing ... 193

7 **Expansion and Integration: Trauma Release
During the Perinatal Period** 200
The Nature and Timing of Somatic Trauma
Treatment 200
The Cyclical Nature of Maternal Trauma
Healing 202
Releasing Maternal Trauma Through
Expansion of Experiential Capacity 204
Using Sensory Awareness Skills to Process
Traumatic Memories 207
Working with Specific Forms of Perinatal
Trauma 208
   Traumatic Childbirth 208
   Pregnancy and Infant Loss 211
   Childhood Maltreatment and Abuse 213
Clinical Vignette: Sarah's Integration of
Deadness and Aliveness 214

8 **Making Maternal Healing Whole with
Clinical Creativity and Biopsychosocial
Somatic Treatment Planning** 224
Trauma-Responsive Treatment Planning and
Biopsychosocial Clinical Creativity 224
Treatment Strategy: The Maternal Bodyfulness
Cycle of Empowerment 227
Perinatal Trauma Psychoeducation 229

Referral Considerations for Anti-Inflammatory
Care 233
Treatment Goals and Objectives 234

Appendices 238
Appendix A: Trauma-Informed Intake
Questionnaire for New Mothers/Parents 238
Appendix B: Somatic Self-Regulation Skills
and Exercises 243

Index 245

List of Figures and Tables

Figures

2.1	Causal Loops of Trauma and PMADs	86
4.1	Integrative Model of Somatic Maternal Healing	140
4.2	Main Problem Areas	141
4.3	Maternal Bodyfulness	143
4.4	Therapeutic Phases of Building Maternal Sensory Awareness and Vocabulary	146
6.1	Foundations of Sensory Awareness	182
7.1	Expansive Model of Somatic Maternal Healing	207
8.1	The Maternal Bodyfulness Cycle of Empowerment	229
8.2	Referral Considerations for Anti-Inflammatory Care	234

Tables

0.1	Application of SAMHSA's Principles of Trauma-Informed Care in Somatic Maternal Healing	46
3.1	Aspects of Maternal Bodylessness	106
6.1	Somatic Self-Regulation Skills	190
6.2	Sensation Words	194
6.3	Themes and Reflection Questions for Cultivating Maternal Bodyfulness	196
7.1	Sensory Awareness Skills for Flashbacks	209
8.1	Topics for Psychoeducation	231
8.2	Short-Term and Long-Term Treatment Goals	235

Acknowledgments

I am first and foremost humbled with gratitude for all the women and parents I have worked with in their perinatal transitions and healing journeys.

I am also beholden to express deep and full-bodied gratitude to the following people, who have granted me invaluable forms of inspiration, insight, guidance, support, ideas, feedback, critique, challenges, and encouragement.

Susie Orbach, for all your fierce trail-blazing that paved the way for us to do this work.

Jessica Benjamin, for your unrelenting and paradigm-shifting work to bring mothers out of the shadow of othering.

Andrea O'Reilly, for being a magnificent maternal thinker, scholar, activist, and pioneer, and a most valued voice of wisdom in my "inner chorus" of mothers.

Karen Kleiman, for your pioneering dedication to our field and the invaluable space you hold for our community of Maternal Mental Health professionals.

Christine Caldwell, for your unyielding faith in the body and your wise guidance on how to come back to it.

Kathleen Kendall-Tackett, for your rigorous expertise, impeccable scholarship, and superb editing.

Hillary Walker and all the therapist-moms from the Postpartum Stress Center's support group, for holding a unique and most needed space for the multi-layered experience of mothering while being a perinatal therapist.

Peter Levine, Abi Blakeslee, Glyndie Nickerson, Raja Selvam, Joshua Sylvae, Cindy Brooks, Mahshid Hager, all the amazing SE assistants, and all my SE training "siblings". The entire SE community is a unique and vibrant gift of healing to the world.

Bethany Saltman, without your guidance, this project would never have come true. Your teachings gave me directions and discipline that forever changed my relationship with writing.

Kimberly Ann Johnson, for believing in my project, for instilling jaguar courage to be ambitious, and for being a prime role model for women and mothers on how to live an authentically embodied life of healing.

Molly Caro May, for your radical life-changing teachings that made me trust in brilliance, and for being the midwife to my body stories.

To all the Birth Yourself workshop mamas and The Loam Dwellers, for offering yourselves to the interweaving of our body stories across the world.

Gabrielle Kaufman, my dearest wise mentor, for your unrelenting support and encouragement and for calling and guiding me into this work without hesitation.

To all my wonderful colleagues at Maternal Mental Health NOW, for your fierce dedication to this work, your energies nurture me.

Wendy Davis, for being an inspiring maternal figure of leadership in our family of the Perinatal Mental Health community.

Lorinda Peterson, for the excellent feedback and editing.

Jodi Pawluski, for crucial guidance, feedback, and encouragement.

Erin Iwanusa, for your inspiring and encouraging dedication to healing in the perinatal field.

Bianca Martinez, for your sensitive and knowledgeable support.

Robin Roberts, for carefully and skillfully guiding my nervous system through many intense waves of my reproductive journey.

JoAnn Culbert-Koehn, for helping me through the cauldron of the maternal transition with your courage and encouragement.

Kelly Baker, for holding space for me in the most nurturing way and helping me stay committed to the work with your unapologetic, creative, and subversive force.

Bridget Cross, for showing me how to alchemize perinatal rage into the gold of healing, for inspiring me deeply by extending your heart during times of much postpartum upheaval, for your endless patience and poignant feedback, and for your friendship.

Camilla Lærke Mors, for dit uendelige hjerte.

Carol Marks, for delivering me the message of the calling to take the journey of somatic healing, on top of all the precious wisdom you were already sharing with me.

My networking group of Maternal Studies Scholars, for always offering me insightful stimulation and inspiration for the most overlooked and most underrated topic of philosophic inquiry.

My husband and children, for being the best people imaginable to make life with.

List of Abbreviations

PMAD	Perinatal Mood and Anxiety Disorder
PPD	Postpartum Depression
PPA	Postpartum Anxiety
PTSD	Post-Traumatic Stress Disorder
PTSS	Post-Traumatic Stress Symptoms
TIC	Trauma-Informed Care

Introduction
Why We Need Maternal Healing that Includes Self, Body, and Society

When I became a mother in the early Spring of 2012, it felt like I walked through a big, heavy door that then slammed shut behind me. This isn't only a metaphor for my emotional experience of my transition to motherhood; it was also a physical experience. Sudden and intense vibrations were traveling through my body, like those felt when a door slams behind you. Everything was shaking and vibrating in my body and nervous system. It was a panicked feeling like having been locked out, only not from a house, but from any sense of safety and certainty of myself as a body in the world, the way I was used to. There was no locksmith to call to get back in, which made me acutely aware of my towering despair about the new responsibility for my newborn. Back then, I understood that my feelings reflected the magnitude of becoming a parent on an emotional level. Today I also understand that the experience was reflective of the unique clash of the transformations of the nervous system and body that takes place in the transition to motherhood and having survived a traumatic birth that cut into the deepest layers of my interpersonal history and attachment trauma. We say that becoming a parent will open one's heart. We don't talk as much about how parenthood will also open one's body and nervous system, especially if one goes through pregnancy and childbirth carrying any amount of trauma.

I call this physical transformation a "nervous system expansion" of motherhood, although it can often feel the opposite. It can feel like an uprooting or an upheaval, like being floored, disheveled, or fragmented, especially if one's nervous system lodges traumatic wounds and dysregulating memories. But namely, because it is an expansion, becoming a parent is a unique opportunity for healing those wounds. It is an expansion because it is a development of the new mother's nervous system that enables her to coregulate in ways that her newborn needs to survive and develop. I also call it an expansion because of my belief that healing of trauma in the perinatal period is not only possible but that the transition to parenthood holds a particular potential for transformative healing. The expansion into the coregulating field of the postpartum phase is indeed what offers the unique potential for healing. But this potential for healing can only be fully unlocked by bringing the body into the process. I did not realize this until years after I became a mother when I began training in Somatic Experiencing®, a body-based trauma resolution model.

The maternal transition is an expansion from a psycho-biological evolutionary perspective of the nervous system, although it comes with acute vulnerabilities. The evolutionary forces of reproduction and caring for our children are some of the strongest forces we experience in our bodies if we become parents. Adaptive processes elicited by reproduction are inherently constructive; new capacities are formed by the new need to take care of our young. I also call it an expansion for psychological and trauma-informed reasons: Transitioning to parenthood is a development of the self that must be acknowledged as more than a "developmental crisis", as classic psychoanalysis described the psychological process of becoming a mother. It is more than an adjustment or a role transition, although it is also that. I see the transition to parenthood as one of the most significant transformations in human lifespan development.

Returning to the shell-shocked newborn mother sitting in the middle of the night with her newborn in her arms. She appeared on the outside to be physically stable, from a medical standpoint. Her baby was fine, she was medically stable. But internally, her nervous system was a dark ocean of dysregulation and overwhelm, a concoction of old and new trauma circuiting her new maternal nervous system. What do you do when a new mother like her walks into your office? Or shows up on your telehealth screen? How do you sit through a session with her, in your own body? How does your nervous system respond to the ocean of dysregulation she is carrying? How do you even begin to help her? Several times I experienced sitting across from providers who wanted to help me but were clearly too overwhelmed in their own nervous systems by my very presence and internal state of chaos. My training in somatic trauma treatment helped me realize that no amount of cognitive talk therapy could have given me what I needed at that time.

Since I started specializing in Maternal Mental Health and trauma treatment, these questions have been presenting themselves and demanding answers. My process of taking on these questions, both as a clinician receiving that new mother in my practice and as having been that mother myself, and my somatic training, lead me to write this book. How do we sit with new mothers and parents who are shaking to their core? How do we help them navigate their transition to parenthood when it was either traumatic, reactivated their previous trauma, or both? How can we make sure that we will not let our own fears and overwhelm keep us from entering the relational work that the new mother or parent in front of us needs?

My work with these questions and my somatic training led me to create a biopsychosocial framework and psychotherapy approach to Maternal Mental Health that is not just trauma-informed, but also trauma-responsive through the integration of somatic therapy. As research has demonstrated that multiple biological, psychological, and societal factors are at play and interact in Perinatal Mood and Anxiety Disorders (PMADs) (Yim et al., 2015), an interdisciplinary approach is therefore required to fully understand their etiology (Barba-Müller et al., 2019). We also now realize that perinatal clients are not a homogeneous clinical group (Vanwetswinkel et al., 2022). Furthermore, understanding Maternal Mental Health requires consideration of the sociopolitical contexts (Fisher et al., 2018). Maternal Mental Health is thus a field that requires *biopsychosocially oriented clinical practice* (term by Borrell-Carrió et al., 2004) and trauma-focused interventions. Advances in neuroscience and psychoneuroimmunology, the study of biological stress responses, have been crucial in shedding light on the complex links between trauma, stress, inflammatory responses, and postpartum depression (Kendall-Tackett, 2017). With these new insights, we can avoid both the over-simplifying explanations of PMADs being caused solely by reproductive hormonal changes and the reductionistic idea that the answer to a woman's Mental Health issues in her maternal transition is found only in her individual psychological history. A woman's attachment and interpersonal history are indeed important for understanding her experience of the maternal transition, but contemporary feminist psychoanalysis offers a crucial critique of the classic psychoanalytic model that failed to acknowledge her full subjectivity as a mother. Furthermore, Maternal Mental Health is a field with significant and deeply concerning disparities making it an urgent necessity to understand and target psychosocial and systemic aspects. The disparities in both Maternal Health and Maternal Mental Health reflect the racial and economic fault lines of the world. The American College of Obstetrics and Gynecology (2020) has stated that "[s]ystemic and institutional racism are pervasive in our country and in our country's health care institutions, including the fields of obstetrics and gynecology." It is deeply concerning that research continues to demonstrate that women of color and their children experience disproportionately higher rates of maternal and neonatal mortality and morbidity (White et al., 2022). The sociopolitical and cultural contexts women in the perinatal period are immersed in influence the conceptual frameworks of Maternal Mental Health care (Fisher et al., 2018). We live in a time of increasing awareness of the wide-ranging impacts of trauma in both the clinical professional world and society at large. *Somatic Maternal Healing* is built on an appreciation of how a trauma-focused perspective continually reveals the complex interactions between biological, psychological, and social factors – and continually points us towards trauma-responsive interventions that address all three levels.

A trauma-informed biopsychosocial approach shows us that we cannot draw solely from one area of research or one treatment modality if we are to effectively address the current public health crisis in Maternal Mental Health. *Somatic Maternal Healing* integrates three schools of psychology to treat perinatal trauma: Feminist psychoanalytic theory and practice to address interpersonal and intersubjective aspects (issues related to maternal embodied subjectivity), somatic psychology and psychobiology and clinical techniques to address the physical aspects (nervous system changes, trauma biology, anxiety, affect regulation, dysregulation, and coregulation), and matricentric feminism to address the social and systemic issues (harmful ideologies of motherhood that impact systems of care and cultural discourses). These approaches overlap, critique, challenge, and supplement each other. What I discovered is that each approach, in its own way, points to the importance of the body. For many forms of perinatal trauma, like traumatic childbirth, pregnancy loss, mothering as an abuse survivor, or reproductive medical complications, the body is the site of the trauma. At the same time, the body is undergoing profound changes and sensory reorganization during the maternal transition that require extensive attention and care. A mother is subjected to constant projections from her surroundings directed at her new corporeality; her body being the concretization of her new caregiving role and relationship with her baby. Further, the new mother is first and foremost mothering from and with her body, in the decidedly nonverbal visceral coregulatory realm of caring for her infant. Not including the body in Maternal Mental Health seems both illogical and unwise.

From the psychodynamic approach, contemporary feminist psychoanalysis shows us that becoming and being a maternal subject is fraught with conflict and a destabilization of the embodied sense of self, which is both exacerbated by and intertwined with trauma. Medical and Health Psychology research shows that the delicate biology of reproduction interacts with the biology of trauma and stress, making the perinatal transition a time of heightened biological vulnerability, yet also a time of plasticity and opportunity for healing. Matricentric feminist theory and research offer critiques of culturally based ideologies of motherhood, demonstrating how patriarchal and institutionalized motherhood ideology produces discriminatory and harmful cultural narratives. My belief is that we must draw on and integrate knowledge from all these paradigms in our clinical work if we are to make Maternal Mental Health fully trauma-responsive. *Somatic Maternal Healing* is an approach that targets the psychological, biological, and psychosocial levels simultaneously.

With the knowledge of how subjectivity is destabilized and impacted by trauma in the maternal transition, causing an experience of disconnect called bodylessness (Caldwell, 2018a), we discover how it can be reclaimed through the embodied assertion of a new sense of self and how this is crucial to the trauma healing process. The postpartum state may create a sense of self-loss, but it can be balanced by an embodied experience of claiming one's new maternal self. I call this maternal bodyfulness; a development of Caldwell's (2018a) concept of bodyfulness. Maternal bodyfulness is the antidote to the forms of bodylessness that are particular to the perinatal period: It is the cultivation of a deeper experiential and reflective knowledge of one's embodied subjectivity as a mother where mothering is discovered as an expression of self as opposed to a role prescribed by cultural expectations. Our growing knowledge about the biology of reproduction, Maternal Mental Health, and how they link to resilience calls us to acknowledge both the vulnerabilities and the opportunities of the perinatal transition and seize the promising opportunities for interrupting the depression-inducing vicious cycles of inflammatory responses to trauma and stress through holistic anti-inflammatory interventions. Emerging research on maternal brain development corroborates this call for a shift from a focus on only the vulnerabilities towards acknowledgment of the opportunities for growth and healing of the perinatal transition through coregulatory interventions. Finally, feminist analysis of current mothering ideologies reveals the overarching systemic issues of oppressive and discriminatory norms contributing to the disparities in Maternal Mental Health.

Matricentric feminist analysis and research have demonstrated that social discourses on motherhood convey dictates for normative mothering that cause harm by being unrealistic and unattainable for all mothers and especially those who do not – or will not – live up to these standards (O'Reilly, 2021). We are thus urged to see that our work with the assertion of the diversity of maternal subjectivities is not limited to the individual realm but reaches into psychosocial discourses and community activism that fight harmful systems. The good news here is that actively resisting the oppressive narratives of institutionalized motherhood can make mothering an empowering experience. Combining all these approaches encourages biopsychosocial thinking that challenges the single-disciplinary tunnel vision of the medical model and dogmatic psychoanalysis and the lack of systemic psychosocial activism perspectives in clinical psychology. Matricentric feminism has enabled me to expand my clinical model to a framework that centers on the empowerment of mothers. This feels monumental in light of the problematic history of how clinical psychology and psychiatry have participated (and in some ways still participate) in the oppressive dynamics of patriarchal motherhood and intensive mothering ideology.

Several studies have confirmed that rates of PMADs rose during the COVID-19 pandemic (Bajaj et al., 2022; Chen et al., 2022). Mental health issues for women in the perinatal period were already recognized as a growing public health concern before the pandemic (National Institute of Mental Health, 2020). It is no surprise that the world of Maternal Mental Health is undergoing significant developments these years. We are seeing legislation for screening protocols and the implementation of collaborative models across systems of care. Since 2015 there has been an increase in federal and state legislation in the U.S. focusing on Maternal Mental Health, for example, the Bringing Postpartum Depression Out of the Shadows Act of 2015 and the 21st Century Cures Act, which included support for identification and treatment of maternal depression. In California, Assembly Bill 2193 passed in 2018, requiring providers to screen for perinatal mood disorders and ordering health insurers to develop Maternal Mental Health programs that promote quality and cost-effectiveness. Specialized reproductive psychiatric care ensures that medications can be safely and sensibly used by pregnant and breastfeeding mothers in dire need of them, and new medication options are being developed (e.g., Zulresso). Postpartum Support International launched the first international certification for Perinatal Mental Health in 2018. The need for effective treatment of PMADs continues to be present: At least 20% of mothers experience anxiety and/or depression with an even higher prevalence among women of color. Even more concerning is the research indicating that up to 50% of women with symptoms of PMADs do not receive treatment. The prevalence range for PTSD in the postpartum period ranges from 4% to as high as 17% for high-risk groups (Grisbrook & Letourneau, 2021). But not meeting the criteria for the PTSD diagnosis does not mean the absence of trauma; symptoms of traumatic stress after childbirth fall along a continuum of varying degrees of reactions that impact functioning and the adjustment to motherhood (Fisher et al., 2018). Trauma is identified as a major factor in Perinatal Mental Health (Seng & Taylor, 2015). We are living in a time of trauma awareness awakening in clinical psychology and in the wider societal discourses where the advancements of trauma research from the last 30–40 years are increasingly integrated across paradigms and disciplines.

The options for top-down psychotherapy treatment of PMADs are abounding, for example, iterations of Interpersonal Psychotherapy and Cognitive-Behavioral Therapy specifically for the treatment of PMADs. They are, however, not trauma-focused or bottom-up modalities. A promising perinatal adaptation of EMDR has also emerged (Chiorino et al., 2020), which is a protocol-based trauma-focused bottom-up modality. And yet there are no established biopsychosocial clinical frameworks for Maternal Mental Health that integrate a wide range of somatic trauma treatment techniques with psychodynamic and feminist thinking specifically for this population. Psychotherapists working with new mothers currently do not have access to a treatment model that fully integrates: 1. somatic trauma treatment informed by interpersonal neurobiology and 2. women-centered and culturally focused schools of therapy that address cultural bias issues inherent in both traditional psychoanalysis and cultural norms for motherhood. This is highly problematic given that an increasing amount of research is showing that trauma and systemic cultural contexts are significant factors in Maternal Mental Health (Fisher et al., 2018; Seng & Taylor, 2015), and a similarly increasing amount of research is showing that somatic or bottom-up approaches are crucial for effective trauma treatment (Schore, 2021). The current literature on evidence-based models for the treatment of trauma is characterized by a glaring absence of studies that include pregnant women (Nillni et al., 2018) and very few studies that include postpartum women (Vesel & Nickasch, 2015), most of these focusing on top-down modalities. Expecting and new mothers have unique needs and vulnerabilities that differ from the general population. We need a trauma treatment model for the perinatal population that is developed around these unique needs.

We have an abundance of research from developmental psychology demonstrating that attachment development is a somatic and experiential phenomenon of coregulation of the nervous systems of infants and caregivers (Schore, 2021). My somatic approach is not only motivated by a trauma perspective, but also by the insights from developmental psychology that demonstrate that working with any new parent is to work within the early attachment matrix. However, this book will not include an overview or discussion of the nature of early development and attachment from the infant's perspective. There is plenty of high-quality literature available on this. This book is fully dedicated to the mother's perspective and her healing process in psychotherapy from a trauma-informed and feminist psychology approach.

I deliberately use the terms Maternal (or Parental) Mental Health because I see a confluence of the term "perinatal" with "early child development". The field of Perinatal Psychology is not synonymous with Perinatal Mental Health which can cause confusion. The growing awareness of the term "perinatal" (literal meaning is "pertaining to the period immediately before and after birth") has contributed to the preponderance of focus on the child's perspective and issues related to child development and – concerningly – this is happening at the expense of focusing on the mother's or parent's perspective. Although we cannot separate infant and parental mental health, there are urgent reasons why it is crucial to establish a clinical field and treatment modalities dedicated specifically to the maternal experience. Contemporary feminist developments of psychodynamic theory, informed by rigorous parent-infant and attachment research, have shown us that mothers and parents are not merely "objects" or attachment figures who fulfill certain caregiver functions for the child but subjects in their own right. But being the proto-typical other and the fleshy landscape of our primal non-verbal emergent self-state, the maternal subject is someone we all struggle to truly acknowledge as a subject. Mothers disrupt our sense of what it means to be a subject. In feminist psychoanalysis and philosophy, we find valuable analyses of these epistemological paradoxes and problems and their consequences in the world. One of the most influential voices of modern relational psychoanalysis, Jessica Benjamin (1988) points out that "the child has a need to see the mother, too, as an independent subject, not simply as the 'external world'" (p. 23) and that "denial of the mother's subjectivity, in theory and in practice, profoundly impedes our ability to see the world as inhabited by equal subjects." (1995, p. 31). Benjamin's work is informed by decades of mother-infant observational research (e.g., Beebe & Lachmann, 1988). Asserting the mother's perspective is not only about distinguishing the clinical specialization of Maternal Mental Health from other specializations, but about addressing the very problems that the erasure of her perspective causes. When Maternal Mental Health is drowned out in the contexts of seemingly enveloping fields like Perinatal Psychology, Attachment Theory, and Family and Infant Mental Health, we lose the distinct emphasis on the mother's perspective that we need to deeply appreciate if we are to help her heal from trauma by claiming her maternal subjectivity in an embodied way and fight the psychosocial structures and dynamics that perpetuate her suffering.

This book is for clinicians of all kinds and anyone working relationally with expecting and new mothers and families. It is written from my belief in the value of theoretical diversity, integrative thinking, and clinical creativity. It also assumes the understanding of interpersonal neurobiology that the essence of psychotherapy lies in nonverbal affective relational dynamics (Schore, 2012). We need non-dogmatic treatment models; a strictly classic psychoanalytic approach will not adequately address the somatic aspects of trauma treatment in the perinatal context, and a somatic technique on its own will not fully include the crucial psychosocial discussions related to the cultural factors relevant to Maternal Mental Health. In my development of this framework, I have identified the following rationale for emphasizing a somatic approach in Perinatal Mental Health:

- ◆ Trauma and traumatic stressors are significant risk factors for PMADs – somatic bottom-up approaches are important and effective for trauma treatment.
- ◆ Harmful unrealistic standards for mothering in societal discourses, ethnic disparities, and health inequity are all acute concerns in Maternal Mental Health and interlink with trauma factors – a culturally focused somatic approach can address this connection. Being trauma-informed is a prerequisite for cultural and diversity humility – and being trauma-informed means being body-informed.
- ◆ New parents are building attachments with their babies, in the "coregulation field" – somatic approaches address regulation and coregulation, which is crucial for that relational development, both the infant's development and that of the new parental identity and role. The biopsychosocial adaptations of the perinatal period make it a time of heightened vulnerable to trauma, but it also offers a unique opportunity for deeper relational trauma healing work. This potential can only be fully unlocked if the body is brought into the treatment through a focus on coregulation.

Regarding work in the coregulating field of the mother-infant dyad, the illusion that a mother can magically "know" her baby intuitively is problematic. While intuitive feelings and insights are indeed important to look at in maternal identity development, forming an attachment to a baby is concretely a complex and intense bodily experience and work of constant coregulation of two new and raw nervous systems. There is no by-passing this process; the work of coregulation. This physicality of mother-work must not only be acknowledged in therapeutic work with mothers, but actively used as the curative venue for intervention. Becoming a mother is to be born again, so in a sense, the mother is a newborn too, and therefore in acute need of being mothered herself. The new mother's nervous system is "newborn" in the sense of the expansion and transformation that having a baby will do to the body – and must be cared for and responded to from that perspective. Babies make a mess, as do bodies. Especially the reproductive bodily processes. Attachment-building and trauma healing are "messy" processes. A somatic approach is needed to adequately address this "messiness".

Asserting one's bodily integrity is part of the maternal transition. Due to contemporary developments in mainstream media culture related to body image, we see new complex challenges for women navigating the body transformations of motherhood. We are seeing new discourses related to female body ownership, societal views on female embodiment and bodily meanings, and somatic expressions. Some of these changes are liberating, but some also pose challenges for mothers. The pressure to achieve a certain body outcome after pregnancy has been intensified through celebrity culture and has women engaging in the "body work" of maintaining certain maternal bodily standards (O'Brien Hallstein, 2015). Parenting is not an achievement or a performance. It's a unique relationship of love and meaning. Mothering should never be judged as a performance because it does not make sense to view mothering only as a performance, task, or assignment. Mothering is a unique relationship with a child, with and from one's entire self; where meaning and love are continuously co-created by mother and child through intense bodily work of coregulation and nonverbal intersubjective relating. The cultural expectations, norms, and myths that frame mothering as an achievement cause harm, especially when they perpetuate negative bias related to race, gender, SES, sexual orientation, marital status, physical appearance, and other aspects of identity. Affirming mothering as a relational bodyful subjective experience – as opposed to the achievement of living up to the dictates of institutionalized motherhood – requires us to resist and challenge these expectations and myths.

Our bodies tell stories. Maternal bodies tell the stories of maternal transitions and transformations, including their elements of upheaval, pain, and trauma, on personal and cultural political levels. Maternal bodies, especially those that don't fit into the narrow model of normative institutionalized motherhood, are heavily politicized. The stories of the maternal body carry feelings, depth, and vulnerabilities related to the massive transformation of one's embodied subjectivity that becoming a mother involves. I believe therapeutic work with mothers must be acutely tuned in to these maternal body stories and body-related feelings if it is to be truly trauma-responsive and empowering. Maternal Mental Health in the 21st century has become increasingly trauma-informed. However, for Maternal Mental Health to be fully trauma-informed, it must also become body-informed. *Somatic Maternal Healing* is a clinical framework that makes Maternal Mental Health body-informed.

Outline of the Book

The book is presented in two parts. Part I works through the theoretical and research issues that the *Somatic Maternal Healing* model is built on. Part II is the clinical application and techniques that starts with an overview of the key clinical skills and goals.

Part I opens with an introductory overview of the biopsychosocial approach to defining perinatal trauma and understanding trauma symptoms in the context of the perinatal period. It includes a definition of perinatal trauma, an overview of statistics and prevalences, a review of common types of perinatal trauma, and a discussion of manifestations of trauma symptoms in the maternal transition. An overview of the biopsychosocial approach of Somatic Maternal Healing is presented using SAMHSA's principles for trauma-informed care. In line with the biopsychosocial framework, Chapters 1, 2, and 3 are dedicated to the psychological, biomedical, and sociological respectively. Chapter 1 examines how feminist psychoanalytic theories of maternal subjectivity inform clinical work. A crucial contribution from psychodynamic thinking to somatic psychology is the opportunity to understand nervous system reactions and patterns not only as biology, but also as expressions of our complex intersubjective dynamics and the struggles related to recognizing and asserting an embodied sense of subjectivity in the maternal transition. In Chapter 2, I take on the question of the nervous system expansion of motherhood from a trauma and psychoneuroimmunological perspective. A solid body of research on trauma, in general, is established, but trauma must be understood in a different light in relation to the transition to motherhood. Research from psychoneuroimmunology has revealed a range of links between inflammatory and stress responses, trauma, the biology of reproduction, and PMADs. Chapter 3 is dedicated to the psychosocial and systemic aspects at play in the perinatal period and PMADs through the societal critical analysis of institutionalized mothering that mother-focused feminist thinking offers (matricentric feminism). Part I ends with a review and synthesis of the comprehensive research foundation of somatic interventions and how they link to current knowledge about maternal transition and perinatal trauma (Chapter 4).

In Part II, the clinical framework and tools of *Somatic Maternal Healing* are unfolded. In the Introduction to Part II, the principles, main problem areas, treatment goals and strategy, and key clinical skills are presented. Chapter 5 unfolds the relational nature of the work by demonstrating the concept of somatic resonance and how it is adapted for the perinatal period and its transferential field. I will explain the importance of somatic countertransference processing for perinatal therapy. Chapter 6 describes the tools for building sensory awareness and maternal sensory vocabulary, which I call maternal bodyfulness as a development of Caldwell's (2018a) concept of bodyfulness. This is the clinical foundation for facilitating the somatically anchored new maternal self that is needed for subsequent trauma resolution. Chapter 7 presents a strategy for targeted trauma resolution that takes the conditions of mothering into account and allows for the integration of other modalities and clinical techniques. The somatic clinical tools in Chapters 5–7 of this book draw on somatic psychology, including elements of Levine's (2010) model of Somatic Experiencing®, Caldwell's theory of body identity and body narrative (2016), and her concept and practice of bodyfulness (2018a, 2018b), and Orbach's (2006, 2009) psychoanalytic approach to bodily focused intersubjective transference work, particularly her work with somatic countertransference reactions. As *Somatic Maternal Healing* is not protocol-based, but a biopsychosocial framework with clinical tools, it can be adapted to and integrated with other approaches and modalities.

Working with trauma during the perinatal period requires clinical flexibility above all. In Chapter 8, I explain how the clinical process can become creative if we shift from a narrow focus on individual psychotherapy towards the biopsychosocially oriented clinical practice of treatment planning that addresses mind, body, and society. With the overarching principles of resonance and perinatal sensory awareness and vocabulary, options for concrete psychotherapy activities are wide. In addition, the insights from biomedical research and sociocultural critique can be used for advocacy, empowering psychoeducation, and careful referrals, with the individual client's circumstances, trauma history, identity, and psychosocial context in mind. The aim is to engage our clients in a holistic healing process that is more than individual psychotherapy sessions.

Somatic Maternal Healing is an approach founded on the appreciation of mothering as a practice of exploring, discovering, verbalizing, and asserting oneself as a maternal subject in an embodied relational way, intertwined with one's lifelong trauma healing process. It is founded on the belief that mothering can be a practice that is not in opposition or a challenge to trauma healing, but on the contrary conducive to it. When treatment of trauma in the perinatal context is done with an appreciation of the biopsychosocial particularities of the maternal transition, it can make a woman's mothering empowering. My hope is that by reading this book, as a clinician you will feel less apprehension about the tender work of trauma healing in the perinatal period. That you will connect deeper to the "clinical courage" in yourself to hold embodied space for mothers and parents who come to you when they are in dire need of healing, shaken by trauma during one of their most vulnerable life transitions. That you will connect to a felt sense of activism happening in the relational and somatic work of therapy in the perinatal period; activism that pushes back against cultural and systemic inequality and millennia-old oppression of mothers and supports the new mother in claiming her new maternal self in a bodyful way through her healing journey.

References

American College of Obstetricians and Gynecologists et al. (2020). *Joint Statement: Collective Action Addressing Racism.* Retrieved from https://www.acog.org/news/news-articles/2020/08/joint-statementobstetrics-and-gynecology-collective-action-addressing-racism

Bajaj, M.A., Salimgaraev, R., Zhaunova, L., & Payne, J.L. (2022). Rates of self-reported postpartum depressive symptoms in the United States before and after the start of the COVID-19 pandemic. *Journal of Psychiatric Research, 151,* 108–112. 10.1016/j.jpsychires.2022.04.011

Barba-Müller, E., Craddock, S., Carmona, S., & Hoekzema, E. (2019). Brain plasticity in pregnancy and the postpartum period: Links to maternal caregiving and mental health. *Archives of Women's Mental Health, 22,* 289–299. 10.1007/s00737-018-0889-z

Beebe, B., & Lachmann, F. (1988). The contribution of mother-infant mutual influence to the origins of self- and object representations. *Psychoanalytic Psychology, 5,* 305–337. 10.1037/0736-9735.5.4.305

Benjamin, J. (1988). *The bonds of love: Psychoanalysis, feminism, and the problem of domination.* Pantheon Books.

Benjamin, J. (1995). *Like subjects, love objects: Essays on recognition and sexual difference.* University Press.

Borrell-Carrió, F., Suchman, A.L., & Epstein, R.M. (2004). The biopsychosocial model 25 years later: Principles, practice, and scientific inquiry. *Annals of Family Medicine, 2*(6), 576–582. 10.1370/afm.245

Caldwell, C.M. (2016). Body identity development: Definitions and discussions. *Body, Movement and Dance in Psychotherapy, 11*(4), 220–234. 10.1080/17432979.2016.1145141

Caldwell, C.M. (2018a). *Bodyfulness. Somatic practices for presence, empowerment, and waking up in this life*. Shambala Publications.

Caldwell, C.M. (2018b). Body identity development: Who we are and who we become. In C.M. Caldwell, & L.B. Leighton (Eds.), *Oppression and the body. Roots, resistance, and resolutions* (pp. 31–50). North Atlantic Books.

Chen, Q., Li, W., Xiong, J., & Zheng, X. (2022). Prevalence and risk factors associated with postpartum depression during the COVID-19 pandemic: A literature review and meta-analysis. *International Journal of Environmental Research and Public Health*, *19*(4), 2219. 10.3390/ijerph19042219

Chiorino, V., Cattaneo, M.C., Macchi, E.A., Salerno, R., Roveraro, S., Bertolucci, G.G., Mosca, F., Fumagalli, M., Cortinovis, I., Carletto, S., & Fernandez, I. (2020). The EMDR recent birth trauma protocol: A pilot randomised clinical trial after traumatic childbirth. *Psychology & Health*, *35*(7), 795–810. 10.1080/08870446.2019.1699088

Fisher, J., Acton, C., & Rowe, H. (2018). Mental health problems among childbearing women: Historical perspectives and social determinants. In M. Muzik, & K.L. Rosenblum (Eds.), *Motherhood in the face of trauma: Pathways towards healing and growth* (pp. 3–20). Springer. 10.1007/978-3-319-65724-0

Grisbrook, M.A., & Letourneau, N. (2021). Improving maternal postpartum mental health screening guidelines requires assessment of post-traumatic stress disorder. *Canadian Journal of Public Health*, *112*(2), 240–243. 10.17269/s41997-020-00373-8

Kendall-Tackett, K.A. (2017). *Depression in new mothers. Causes, consequences, and treatment alternatives* (3rd ed.). Routledge.

Levine, P.A. (2010). *In an unspoken voice. How the body releases trauma and restores goodness*. North Atlantic Books.

National Institute of Mental Health. (2020). *Perinatal depression*. NIH Publication No. 20-MH-8116. Retrieved from https://www.nimh.nih.gov/health/publications/perinatal-depression

Nillni, Y.I., Mehralizade, A., Mayer, L., & Milanovic, S. (2018). Treatment of depression, anxiety, and trauma-related disorders during the perinatal period: A systematic review. *Clinical Psychology Review*, *66*, 136–148. 10.1016/j.cpr.2018.06.004

O'Brien Hallstein, L. (2015). *Bikini-ready moms. Celebrity profiles, motherhood, and the body*. State University of New York Press.

Orbach, S. (2006). How can we have a body?: Desires and corporeality. *Studies in Gender & Sexuality*, *7*(1), 89–111. 10.2513/s15240657sgs0701_9

Orbach, S. (2009). *Bodies*. Picador.

O'Reilly, A. (2021). *Matricentric feminism. Theory, activism, practice. The 2nd edition*. Demeter Press. 10.2307/j.ctv1k2j331

Schore, A.N. (2012). *The science of the art of psychotherapy*. W.W. Norton.

Schore, A.N. (2021). The interpersonal neurobiology of intersubjectivity. *Frontiers in Psychology*, *12*, 648616. 10.3389/fpsyg.2021.648616

Seng, J., & Taylor, J. (Eds.). (2015). *Trauma informed care and the perinatal period*. Dunedin Academic Press.

Vanwetswinkel, F., Bruffaerts, R., Arif, U., & Hompes, T. (2022). The longitudinal course of depressive symptoms during the perinatal period: A systematic review. *Journal of Affective Disorders*, *315*, 213–223. 10.1016/j.jad.2022.06.087

Vesel, J., & Nickasch, B. (2015). An evidence review and model for prevention and treatment of postpartum posttraumatic stress disorder. *Nursing for Women's Health*, *19*(6), 504–525. 10.1111/1751-486X.12234

White, R.S., & Aaronson, J.A. (2022). Obstetric and perinatal racial and ethnic disparities. *Current Opinion in Anaesthesiology*, *35*(3), 260–266. 10.1097/ACO.0000000000001133

Yim, I.S., Tanner Stapleton, L.R., Guardino, C.M., Hahn Holbrook, J., & Dunkel Schetter, C. (2015). Biological and psychosocial predictors of postpartum depression: Systematic review and call for integration. *Annual Review of Clinical Psychology*, *11*, 99–137. 10.1146/annurev-clinpsy-101414-020426

Introduction to Part I
Overview of Trauma in the Perinatal Period

Defining Traumatic Stress and Trauma

Perinatal care providers must have a robust understanding of trauma and Post-Traumatic Stress Disorder (PTSD) to effectively treat each perinatal client's unique situation and presentation (Granner & Seng, 2021). The American Psychiatric Association (APA) defines trauma as an event or situation that the individual perceives as threatening to an overwhelming extent, whether they experience or witness it directly or indirectly (APA, 2022). I define perinatal trauma as:

> Trauma reactions in response to the stressors that occur during the perinatal transition. These factors interact with the individual parent's biopsychosocial history, the physiological adaptations of reproduction, medical interventions and iatrogenic effects, the subjective experiences of becoming a parent, and the systemic and cultural contexts the parent is embedded in. These interacting factors can each be the source of trauma and can exacerbate each other's impact.

This definition is deliberately wide because of its biopsychosocial foundation and the nature of the perinatal period. I use the term "perinatal" in this definition to emphasize how trauma that impacts expecting and new mothers impacts the perinatal transition of the entire family. Reproductive trauma is unique because it occurs during a highly sensitive life stage where both parents and infants are particularly vulnerable to the impacts of trauma and traumatic stress. Perinatal trauma is also unique in that it is deeply relational due to the intersubjective and coregulating nature of early attachment formation: If something happens to the baby, it can be traumatic to the mother, and vice versa. Perinatal is a term that encompasses both pregnancy and postpartum. While the definition here uses the term "perinatal" to acknowledge the relational and family context of this particular kind of trauma (and can also include all parents besides mothers), the name of this treatment model, *Somatic Maternal Healing*, uses the term "maternal" because it is centered on treating the mother and emphasizes understanding perinatal trauma from her perspective (the importance of the mother's perspective will be elaborated in Chapter 1 and 3).

Somatic approaches to trauma emphasize not only the event itself, but the individual's psychobiological survival-based reactions (Levine, 2010; Maté, 2010; Porges, 2022; van der Kolk, 2015). These approaches broaden the understanding of trauma towards a biopsychosocial model, where context and resultant interactions across systems influence the outcome (Substance Abuse and Mental Health Services Administration (SAMHSA), 2014b). From a somatic approach, trauma reactions are understood in light of all our psychobiological systems of survival, adaptation, self-regulation, and attachment. Of note here is the insight that the psychobiological systems involved in trauma reactions are also foundational to our general sense of goodness, vitality, and connection (Levine, 2010). This connection is crucial for a deeper understanding of trauma, especially in the perinatal context. Any single exposure to a traumatic event is understood in light of its context and timing in the individual's developmental and relational history. SAMHSA's (2014a) definition of trauma emphasizes that trauma consists of two elements besides exposure to a traumatic event: 1) the individual's experience of the event, and 2) its long-lasting adverse effects. In the perinatal context, we must consider the unique relational, biological, and social circumstances of the perinatal women that influence their experience of trauma and the way it impacts them.

Despite developments towards a more holistic and contextual conceptualization of trauma, the diagnostic understanding of trauma has traditionally focused on PTSD diagnosis. Trauma psychology developed based on the belief that traumatic events were highly unusual and unique before recognizing that traumatic events were common experiences, for example, childhood maltreatment or domestic violence (Smith & Freyd, 2014). The diagnostic criteria for PTSD have been revised several times since it was introduced in the DSM in 1980. But four core features remain the same: Experiencing or witnessing a stressful event, re-experiencing symptoms of the event that include nightmares and (or) flashbacks; efforts to avoid situations, places, and people that are reminders of the traumatic event; and hyperarousal symptoms, such as irritability, concentration problems, and sleep disturbances (Sareen, 2014). The criterion for "negative alterations in cognitions and mood" was added in DSM-5.

The unique element of the PTSD diagnosis is that the assumed cause of the disorder, exposure to a threatening event, is included in the diagnostic criteria (Bonde et al., 2022). According to the diagnostic criteria, symptoms must for a month or longer after the exposure to trauma. In contrast, Acute Stress Disorder develops between 3 days and 1 month after exposure. However, the two are connected in that the symptom criteria are similar, and that Acute Stress Disorder is a strong predictor of PTSD (Bonde et al., 2022). PTSD is highly comorbid with other disorders, but is differentiated by the re-experiencing symptoms (Sareen, 2014). PTSD is also associated with suicidal ideation and behavior, depression, anxiety, medical comorbidities, such as chronic pain, diabetes, and metabolic syndrome, heart diseases, and issues with self-awareness and affect regulation (van de Kamp et al., 2019). Not surprisingly, PTSD is considered a prevalent public health concern (Kornfield et al., 2022). It can last for months and has low spontaneous remission rates compared to other conditions (Kuhfuß et al., 2021). However, the diagnostic criteria and clinical picture of the PTSD diagnosis alone are not adequate for trauma-informed care in the perinatal period.

In the general population, the lifetime prevalence of PTSD has been estimated at 10%–12% for women and 5%–6% for men (Olff, 2017). The prevalence of partial PTSD (not all criteria met, but with functional impairment) is estimated to be between 4%–11% (Kornfield et al., 2022). Most people exposed to potentially traumatic events do not develop PTSD and may have other reactions that do not meet PTSD diagnostic criteria (Bonde et al., 2022; Levine, 2010). However, the absence of PTSD does not mean the absence of trauma. Since the PTSD diagnosis was introduced in DSM-III, the question of possible subsyndromal presentations has been introduced since many survivors of trauma do not meet full diagnostic criteria while still being significantly impacted by symptoms (Mylle & Maes, 2004). Partial (pPTSD) or subthreshold PTSD are subclinical presentations that impair functioning while only meeting some diagnostic criteria (Kornfield et al., 2022; Mylle & Maes, 2004). The current diagnostic options for trauma in the DSM are limited and thus problematic. Trauma symptoms that do not meet the criteria for PTSD can be misdiagnosed as depression, anxiety, or other mental illness (SAMHSA, 2014b). PTSD, depression, and anxiety overlap in their symptomatic presentation (Alcorn et al., 2010). For trauma-related conditions, it is necessary to widen the understanding of trauma to include a developmental perspective on the impact of toxic stress (Franke, 2014) and the related concept of allostatic load (Guidi et al., 2021; McEwen & Stellar, 1993).

Another important distinction is between trauma and stress. Levine (2010) has pointed out that all traumatic events are stressful, but not all forms of stress are traumatic. Stress can be positive, tolerable, or toxic (Franke, 2014). Toxic stress is "severe, prolonged, or repetitive adversity with a lack of the necessary nurturance or support of a caregiver to prevent an abnormal stress response" (Franke, 2014, p. 391). Prolonged activation of physical stress systems like cortisol and inflammatory responses can disrupt neuroimmunological systems that increase the risk for adverse health effects (Beck et al., 2013; Franke, 2014). The interactions between these mechanisms and the maternal transition will be discussed in depth in Chapter 2.

The term allostatic load captures a wider understanding of the biopsychosocial impact of toxic and traumatic stress (Guidi et al., 2021). Allostatic load is a cumulative measure of stressors that overwhelm the body's attempts to regain homeostasis (Guidi et al., 2021; McEwen & Stellar, 1993). McEwen and Stellar (1993) introduced this construct to capture the impact of chronic exposure to fluctuating neuroendocrine stress responses. Toxic stress that causes allostatic load plays a role in mood disorders dysregulation, PTSD, and other mental health conditions (Franke, 2014). From a somatic perspective, both trauma and chronic stress are understood as functional dysregulation of subcortical autonomic, limbic, and arousal systems (Payne et al., 2015). Focusing on toxic stress as a precursor to traumatic stress increases providers' attention to the client's context and developmental history which is crucial for a biopsychosocial approach to trauma treatment and particularly relevant for Perinatal Mental Health (Granner & Seng, 2021; Seng & Taylor, 2015). Likewise, the allostatic load is relevant to a trauma-informed biopsychosocial framework because it integrates biomarkers and clinical data, where psychosocial and biological factors interact in complex ways (Guidi et al., 2021).

Trauma and the Perinatal Period

Trauma is intrinsic to Mental Health issues in general but is particularly relevant in the perinatal period. Trauma symptoms have adverse effects on pregnancy, birth outcomes, post-partum Maternal Mental Health, and child development (Kornfield et al, 2022). Stress, trauma, or PTSD symptoms can increase risks for or exacerbate Postpartum Depression (PPD) (Grekin et al., 2017; Seng & Taylor, 2015). Untreated PTSD symptoms present a significant risk factor for postpartum depression (Becker-Sadzio et al., 2020). Up to 20% of women experience some form of PMAD, trauma-related disorder, or psychosis in the perinatal period (O'Hara & Wisner, 2014), and many mothers' sufferings go undiagnosed and therefore untreated. While PTSD and PPD are highly comorbid, perinatal trauma can also occur without depression. In a recent study by Padin et al. (2022), over ten percent of pregnant women screened positive for PTSD without depression. Perinatal PTSD has unique attributes, antecedents, and outcomes compared to non-perinatal PTSD (Vignato et al., 2017).

Women with a trauma history are at risk of retraumatization in the perinatal period (Polmanteer et al., 2019; Seng & Taylor, 2015). Pregnancy, prenatal care, and delivery involve embodied relational experiences that can trigger traumatic memories or cause new trauma that interacts with previous trauma (Ayers et al., 2016; Granner & Seng, 2021). A prime example of this is traumatic childbirth, which can cause a range of rippling consequences, including breastfeeding complications, bonding issues, and relationship issues (Beck et al., 2013). Interestingly, birth is not listed as an overwhelming life experience in the DSM-5. The DSM-5 defines the "postpartum time" as 2–6 weeks after birth (APA, 2022), however, researchers and clinicians widely acknowledge that PMAD symptoms can manifest up to 1 year after birth (O'Hara & Wisner, 2014). Clinicians can use the specifier, "with postpartum onset" as 1–4 weeks after birth (APA, 2022), which most clinicians recognize as inadequate. PTSD stemming from one pregnancy can manifest during a subsequent pregnancy, or become chronic (Martínez-Vazquez et al., 2021). PTSD in the postpartum period is not a specific diagnosis (Martínez-Vazquez et al., 2021), nor does the DSM-5 offer any other trauma diagnosis specific to the perinatal period.

Perinatal depression screening is recommended by the American College of Obstetricians and Gynecologists (ACOG), but there is no recommendation for trauma screening, despite recommendations from researchers (Grisbrook & Letourneau, 2021; Padin et al., 2022). Prenatal PTSD screening remains rare in obstetric settings (Padin et al., 2022). This is problematic because trauma survivors often will not disclose previous trauma (Sachdeva et al., 2022) and practitioners often label women with trauma symptoms as "difficult" or "non-compliant" (Seng et al., 2009). Such labeling can contribute to clients having negative experiences of interacting with healthcare providers.

Context impacts how trauma is experienced, for example, whether it was intentional (such as violence) or unintentional (such as natural disasters) (SAMHSA, 2014b). In the perinatal period, intentional and unintentional acts can interact. For example, a medical emergency of fetal demise during labor might be unavoidable, but insensitive or invasive care in response to the emergency can exacerbate the mother's experience of trauma. While there are many Perinatal Mental Health issues that are outside our control, research has demonstrated that the quality of maternity care is a significant mediating factor in postpartum PTSD (Ayers et al., 2016; Ford & Ayers, 2011; Seng & Taylor, 2015). Thus, there is potential for preventing postpartum PTSD by improving maternity care (Ayers, 2017).

SAMHSA (2014a, 2014b) describes how trauma disrupts daily routines. New parents are already experiencing an inherent disruption of daily life in the adjustments to postpartum life, especially first-time parents. Mothers and families vary widely in their responses to and coping with postpartum adjustments. Symptoms of traumatic stress after childbirth fall along a continuum of varying degrees of reactions that impact functioning and the adjustment to motherhood (Fisher et al., 2018). The life changes associated with having a baby are intense and profound. Because the postpartum phase changes so many aspects of new mothers' daily lives, providers may not recognize that some of their reactions are trauma related.

Quantitative research on PTSD's effect on pregnancy did not emerge before around 2000 (Seng & Taylor, 2015). The prevalence of PTSD during pregnancy is estimated at approximately 8% (Seng et al., 2009), with higher rates for vulnerable groups. The prevalence of partial PTSD is estimated to be higher. For example, it was 28.6% for women who had previous pregnancy complications (Kornfield et al., 2022). Research indicates that women of color with low income are especially at risk for PTSD during pregnancy, but less likely to seek or receive treatment than white women (Kornfield et al., 2022). One study reported that the prevalence of PTSD in Black pregnant women with a history of trauma exposure was in the range of 34%–40% (Kornfield et al., 2022). Seng et al. (2009) conducted a study (known as "the STACY" project) that demonstrated strong variations in rates of PTSD for Black and white mothers (14% versus 3%). The comorbidity of PTSD and depression was 35%

of those meeting criteria for PTSD in pregnancy. The prevalence of PTSD in the postpartum period is estimated to be at 8% (Verrault et al., 2012), with a range of 4%–17% with higher rates for vulnerable groups (Grisbrook & Letourneau, 2021). Approximately 6% of those cases of postpartum PTSD emerge as a result of childbirth (Ayers et al., 2015a). A study from 2013 by Seng et al. indicated that lifetime PTSD was a stronger predictor of PPD than antenatal depression. Research has also demonstrated that subclinical levels of PSTD impact perinatal women, possibly impacting maternal-infant bonding (Ayers et al., 2006). Despite the robust data on the public health issues of PTSD and trauma-related conditions in women in the perinatal period, treatment studies on trauma-related disorders remain scarce (Nillni et al., 2018).

Types of Perinatal Trauma

Perinatal women can experience many forms of trauma. Some of the most salient trauma exposures are a mother's history of adverse childhood experiences (Choi & Sikkema, 2016), traumatic childbirth (Beck et al., 2013), history of pregnancy loss (Séjourné & Goutaudier, 2020), and history of sexual abuse (Ayers et al., 2016; Granner & Seng, 2021).

Childhood Maltreatment

Seng et al. (2009) examined mothers' trauma histories and found childhood maltreatment significantly increased the risk of pregnancy PTSD. Childhood maltreatment (abuse or neglect of minors) includes physical and/or emotional ill-treatment, sexual abuse, neglect, negligence, and commercial or other exploitation (Souch et al., 2022). A woman's history of child maltreatment can influence attachment development and children's later psychological and physiological wellbeing, including autonomic nervous system functioning (Jokić et al., 2022; Schore, 2013). Insecure mother-infant attachment increases the risk for many serious sequelae in adults including depression and PTSD (Levine, 2010). It is therefore not surprising that research confirms that women with a history of childhood maltreatment are particularly vulnerable to the stress of the perinatal period (Morelen et al., 2018; Souch et al., 2022). Indeed, childhood maltreatment is a significant risk factor for pregnancy PTSD (Cook et al., 2018), and depression and anxiety postpartum (Polmanteer et al., 2019). Cumulative sociodemographic factors, such as income and education, exacerbate risk (Seng et al., 2009). A systematic review by Choi and Sikkema (2016) demonstrated that childhood maltreatment predicts anxiety and depression above and beyond the effects of sociodemographic factors, existing psychopathology, and other life adversities, operating through psychiatric, social, cognitive, and psychobiological pathways that "become especially salient in the perinatal period" (Choi & Sikkema, 2016, p. 427).

Preterm Delivery

Depression, anxiety, or PTSD during pregnancy increases the risks of adverse birth outcomes like low birth weight, preterm birth, and reduced gestational age (Guintivano et al., 2018; Sanjuan et al., 2021). Preterm delivery is a significant form of traumatic birth for both parents and infants. While there are many complex etiologies at play in preterm birth, it is clearly linked to stress and depression (Guintivano et al., 2018). The physiologic underpinnings of PTSD, specifically heightened or dysregulated arousal and inflammation, contribute to adverse pregnancy and birth outcomes (Kornfield et al., 2022). One study indicated that pregnancy PTSD presents a two-fold risk of preterm delivery (Yonkers et al., 2014). Another study showed that women with MDD and PTSD had more than a four-fold increased risk of preterm birth (Guintivano et al., 2018). Untreated depression during pregnancy is associated with a significantly higher risk of preterm birth compared to women without depression, with an even higher risk for women with severe depression (Guintivano et al., 2018).

Traumatic Childbirth and Iatrogenic Effects of Obstetric Care

Traumatic childbirth is unique in that it involves a normal bodily process that has profound psychological and cultural meanings with risks of physical complications and intense emotional distress (Greenfield et al., 2016). There can also be iatrogenic risks from invasive medical procedures (Beck et al., 2013). SAMHSA (2014a) acknowledges the use of invasive medical procedures as potentially re-traumatizing for individuals with a trauma history, but they can also cause trauma in women with no trauma history. Not all women who experience their birth as traumatic develop PTSD (Beck et al., 2013). Traumatic childbirth is a risk factor for PPD comparable to prenatal anxiety and depression (Waller et al., 2022). Factors related to delivery that has been associated with client-reported traumatic childbirth include cesarean birth, greater blood loss, and preterm birth (Waller et al., 2022). Negative events during birth like obstetric complications, emergency cesarean, or prematurity are common, but do not determine that the mother develops postpartum PTSD, however, mothers who do develop postpartum PTSD invariably experience such events during their delivery (Alcorn et al., 2010). Subjective and interpersonal factors are salient, such as when the mother experiences her providers as incompetent or uncaring (Creedy et al., 2000). Low provider support predicts postpartum posttraumatic stress symptoms in women who have a history of trauma (Ford & Ayers, 2011). Trauma history can also negatively impact treatment engagement in the perinatal period (Sachdeva et al., 2022). Even normal perinatal care includes elements that can trigger trauma, such as unwelcome touch, supine position, physical exposure, uncontrolled pain, and lack of control (Granner & Seng, 2021).

Traumatic childbirth includes a range of negative reactions to giving birth where physical trauma like medical injuries may or may not be involved (Greenfield et al., 2016). While the prior history of trauma is a significant risk factor, 6.3% of women with no trauma history had developed birth-related PTSD by week 12 in a study by Alcorn et al. (2010), which demonstrated that childbirth can be a PTSD-inducing event in itself. Traumatic childbirth can lead to posttraumatic stress symptoms (PTSS) or full PTSD (Delicate et al., 2020). Studies on the prevalence of childbirth-related PTSD have been challenged by methodological issues (Alcorn et al., 2010). Birth trauma is often used interchangeably for PTSS and PTSD (Delicate et al., 2020). Research suggests approximately 20%–40% of women report their birth as traumatic (Alcorn et al., 2010; Creedy et al., 2000). Systematic reviews have shown that as many as 16.8% of women experience PTSS after birth such as reexperiencing, hyperarousal, avoidance, and negative alterations to cognition (Delicate et al., 2020).

Beck (2004), a major researcher in the field, defines birth trauma as "an event occurring during the labor and delivery process that involves actual or threatened serious injury or death to the mother or her infant" (p. 28) or "where the woman perceives she is stripped of her dignity" (Beck et al., 2013, p. 8). This definition is based on research that shows that common themes in women's experiences of traumatic childbirth are being stripped of their dignity, feeling not cared for, that providers failed to communicate with them, feelings of powerlessness, exposure, and lack of control, having their experience be dismissed or ignored, feeling abandoned, betrayed, and lonely, and feeling disconnected from their baby and partners (Beck et al., 2013). Beck's research (2011) demonstrates the long-term consequences of traumatic childbirth, including the ripple effects of trauma on breastfeeding, subsequent childbirths, birth anniversary, and mother-infant interaction.

Pregnancy and Infant Loss and Stillbirth

Miscarriage, defined as a pregnancy loss before 20 weeks gestation (Giannandrea et al., 2013), is common; rates are estimated as high as one in four pregnancies (Séjourné & Goutaudier, 2020). Pregnancy loss and stillbirth, defined as pregnancy loss after 20 weeks gestation occurs in approximately one in 100 pregnancies in the US (MacDorman & Gregory, 2015). Infant loss is defined as the loss of a baby who dies within the first year of life. The U.S. infant mortality rate was 5.42 per 1,000 live births in 2020 (Ely & Driscoll, 2022). Regardless of timing, all pregnancy and infant losses are significant stressors and associated with increased risk of PMADs and PTSD, especially in subsequent pregnancies and postpartum. Women with multiple losses are at increased risk compared to women with a single loss (Giannandrea et al., 2013). In a study with 377 bereaved mothers and 232 mothers with live births, bereaved women had four times the risk of depression and seven times the risk of PTSD (Gold et al., 2016). A systematic review demonstrated that mothers who experience stillbirth have a significantly higher risk of depression, anxiety, partial and full PTSD, and full PTSD compared with mothers with live births, and that these issues can persist for years after the loss occurred (Westby et al., 2021).

Risk factors for PTSD after perinatal loss include being single, having no living children, previous psychiatric conditions, lack of support, feelings of responsibility for the loss, and fertility challenges (Séjourné & Goutaudier, 2020). Giannandrea et al. (2013) have argued that pregnancy loss adds to a woman's overall trauma burden and interacts with other trauma.

The quality of care is important for mothers' Mental Health in relation to stillbirth. One study showed that professional support after stillbirth was significantly associated with a decrease in PTSD symptoms (Crawley et al., 2013). Another study showed that women with high social support reported lower levels of re-experiencing symptoms after the stillbirth, indicating that social support can be a protective factor against PTSD (Horsch et al., 2015).

Discrimination and Health Inequity

Discrimination and inequitable care can be another type of trauma impacting perinatal women (Granner & Seng, 2021; Matthews et al., 2021). Higher levels of racial discrimination increase the risk of preterm birth (Guintivano et al., 2018). The rate of preterm birth has declined in recent years, but Black mothers still experience it at a rate 1.5–1.6 times higher than that of White mothers (Braveman et al., 2021). Black women are more likely to be exposed to racial discrimination, and experience psychological stress compared to White women. These factors have been linked to preterm birth (Giurgescu & Misra, 2018). While many factors contribute to the preterm disparity, racial discrimination increases inflammation, which increases the risk of preterm birth

(Braveman et al., 2021). Traumatic stress is also recognized as a likely factor in birth outcome disparities (Seng et al., 2011). One study reported that the prevalence of PTSD in Black pregnant women with a history of trauma exposure ranged from 34% to 40% (Kornfield et al., 2022). Seng et al.'s (2009) study, "the STACY" project, that found rates of PTSD for Black mothers (14%) and White mothers (3%). The comorbidity of PTSD and depression was 35% of those meeting criteria for PTSD in pregnancy.

Women of color are at higher risk for PTSD during pregnancy while simultaneously being less likely to seek or receive treatment than white women (Kornfield et al., 2022). Research also continues to demonstrate that Black mothers and their children experience disproportionately higher rates of maternal and neonatal mortality and morbidity (White et al., 2022). Low-income racial/ethnic minority women have the highest risk for perinatal PTSD given more lifetime exposure to trauma and limited access to mental health care (Kornfield et al, 2022). Lower socioeconomic status alone is associated with a high risk of postpartum depression and pregnancy loss (Giannandrea et al., 2013). Lack of access to quality care contributes to health inequity in perinatal care. Identifying systemic discrimination and health inequity in perinatal mental health is important to shift the blame from individuals to systems (Matthews et al., 2021).

Sexual Abuse

More than 40% of women of childbearing age have experienced some form of sexual violence in their life (Tjaden & Thoennes, 2000), making sexual assault one of the most common forms of trauma for women (Kendall-Tackett, 2017). In the National Violence Against Women (NVAW) Survey, 17.6% of women surveyed reported that they had been the victim of a completed or attempted rape at some time in their life (Tjaden & Thoennes, 2000). Many women go through the perinatal period as sexual abuse survivors and face particular risks (Seng et al., 2009).

A history of sexual trauma is a significant risk factor for birth-related PTSD (Verrault et al., 2012). Sexual abuse history increases the risk for PPD and sleep issues (Swanson et al., 2014). The nature of perinatal care like pelvic exams and obstetric interventions presents a high risk for the reactivation of traumatic memories for sexual abuse survivors (Granner & Seng, 2021; Seng et al., 2009; Sachdeva et al., 2022). Sexual abuse takes many forms but always entails some form of violation of body boundaries. Bodily boundaries and sensory awareness undergo significant rearrangement in the maternal transition.

Intimate Partner Violence (IPV)

IPV is highly traumatogenic and can cause severe dysregulation and stress physiology (Perizzolo Pointet et al., 2018). Partner violence is a common form of violence against women. For example, 64% percent of women who reported being raped, physically assaulted, and/or stalked since age 18 were victimized by a current or former partner (Tjaden & Thoennes, 2000). IPV during the perinatal period is considered a serious public health issue. Some studies indicate that between 3%–9% of women experience abuse during pregnancy, with studies showing rates up to 50% for high-risk groups like low-income single women (Alhusen et al., 2015). A meta-analysis by James et al. (2013) showed that the average reported prevalence of emotional abuse was 28.4%, physical abuse was 13.8%, and sexual abuse was 8%. Risk factors for partner violence during pregnancy include young age, single relationship status, minority race/ethnicity, low income and education, and abuse during a previous pregnancy (Alhusen et al., 2015; James et al., 2013).

IPV during pregnancy is associated with antenatal depression, PPD, and PTSD, often co-occurring (Alhusen et al., 2015). Perizzolo Pointet et al. (2018) found that IPV-PTSD affects several brain functions including socio-emotional processing and emotional appraisal, which are central to parenting. This means mothers with IPV-related PTSD have a "psychobiological disadvantage" related to socio-emotional appraisal in their parenting interactions, where normal mother-child interactions that involve the child being in distress can trigger the mother's trauma symptoms (Perizzolo Pointet et al., 2018).

Disasters and Pandemic Stress

The perinatal period heightens vulnerability to stress, especially in the context of reduced social support (Venta et al., 2021). It is therefore no surprise that rates of postpartum mental illness rose during the COVID-19 pandemic (Bajaj et al., 2022; Chen et al., 2022). Rates of birth trauma also increased (Mayopoulos et al., 2021), likely associated with the increase in stress for maternity care providers (Rao et al., 2021) and restrictions on delivery care and support (Diamond & Colaianni, 2022). These findings align with the significant amount of pre-pandemic literature demonstrating that support during labor and delivery is a crucial factor in birth trauma (Ayers et al., 2015a). A study comparing mothers who gave birth during the COVID-19 pandemic and who developed PTSD with previous studies on childbirth-related PTSD showed higher rates of re-experiencing, avoidance, and hyperarousal (Diamond & Colaianni, 2022).

Many countries separated mothers and newborns to prevent infection. These actions have likely caused more harm than good given that newborns are at very low risk for COVID-related death and that skin-to-skin contact after birth is important for the emotional and physical health of the mother and baby (Rao et al., 2021). A comparative risk analysis demonstrated that the survival benefit of kangaroo mother care far outweighs the risk of death due to COVID-19 for newborns (Minckas et al., 2021). Keeping mothers and newborns together is crucial in maternity care and has been threatened during the pandemic (Rao et al., 2021). This has been particularly harmful to highly vulnerable babies like those born prematurely or with low birth weight who depend on kangaroo mother care (Rao et al., 2021; WHO, 2021). The long-term sequelae of mothers' emotional health from the disruptions of maternity care during the pandemic have yet to be documented.

Trauma Symptoms from a Perinatal Perspective

Trauma impacts our physiology, which means we must carefully consider how trauma symptoms manifest in the perinatal period, a time of significant biopsychosocial changes. Despite research demonstrating that prenatal PTSD increases the risk for perinatal complications, a systematic review concluded that research on prenatal PTSD symptoms, diagnosis, and treatment remains extremely limited (Stevens et al., 2021). Trauma symptoms in the perinatal context are highly complex and require comprehensive and continued assessment and exploration within a safe therapeutic relationship. Social support is a crucial factor in a new mother's distress, so symptom assessment should be considered in light of her current situation of social support. Research on the assessment of trauma in perinatal women presents methodological challenges because normal postpartum symptoms may confound measurements (Ayers et al., 2015b). This is why it is important for clinicians studying the unique conditions of perinatal women to assess trauma using holistic biopsychosocial clinical thinking.

Traumatic experiences are deeply subjective (Levine, 2010). Medicalization of birth can erase women's subjective experiences by focusing solely on the medical outcome of pregnancy, delivery, and recovery (Beck, 2004; Beck et al., 2013). A woman with a healthy baby might have been traumatized by her prenatal care and delivery. In contrast, a woman may have experienced significant obstetric complications but was not traumatized. A woman's history, biology, and social circumstances carry a wide range of risk factors and protective factors that influence whether and how she has trauma reactions and how she experiences them.

One challenge for providers is differentiating between trauma reactions and normal adjustment responses. Overwhelm can be both a natural response to becoming a mother and a trauma symptom. Seng et al. (2010) demonstrated that PTSD-suffering pregnancy women's most frequent symptoms were detachment, loss of interest, anger, and irritability, which can be mistaken for normal reactions to the maternal transition. What differentiates overwhelm from trauma cannot be isolated to single measurable objectives but is a combination of the whole clinical picture of the new mother's functioning. Trauma-related overwhelm makes it hard to take in social support (Porges,

2022) because of the way trauma impacts coregulation functioning and our neurological safety-appraisal system (Porges, 2022; Schore, 2021), which is described in Chapters 4 and 5. The new mother might also have a delayed onset of her trauma reactions and symptoms that can make it hard for her and her surroundings to make sense of them. What follows is an overview of trauma symptoms reviewed from a perinatal perspective.

Delayed Onset

Until recently, PTSD was believed to develop within the first months following trauma exposure. Later research revealed that in 20%–30% of cases, diagnostic criteria are met more than 6 months after exposure (Bonde et al., 2022). PTSS are often heightened for women during pregnancy through 1 year postpartum (Huffphines et al., 2022). Alcorn et al. (2010) demonstrated that assessing for PTSD after the entire first year postpartum showed higher rates than in the early postpartum months, indicating that symptoms can develop later. This is consistent with general research on delayed onset of PTSD. A systemic review by Bonde et al. (2022) showed that few individuals experience asymptomatic delay, and that delayed PTSD is preceded by some PTSD symptoms during the first year in most cases. When defining trauma, SAMHSA (2014a) noted that adverse effects of trauma may have delayed onset. APA's (2013) definition of the postpartum time being 2–6 weeks postpartum is problematic from a trauma-informed perspective. Therapists must carefully consider the delayed-expression specifier as trauma reactions can be delayed following pregnancy, delivery, and the first year after birth. These are eventful transitions, where emotional and nervous system reactions to trauma are easily overlooked or manifest only partially.

The medical focus of prenatal monitoring and anticipation of the delivery, as well as the practicalities of the immediate postpartum phase, will often distract and consume the new mother and those around her. There is little time to pause and carefully assess how the mother is truly feeling and what she is experiencing. She might not be able to recognize her deeper emotional and nervous system reactions just yet. She might be in a state of shock from the intensity of having just met her baby or because she had a traumatic or stressful delivery, or both. Traumatized new mothers can exhibit little to no overt trauma symptoms because they are in survival mode of caring for their newborn, while still experiencing subtle symptoms. Trauma reactions related to medical interventions might be held back by a new mother's freeze response as she depends on continued follow-up care for herself and her baby. The timing of trauma reactions in the perinatal period must be carefully explored considering mothers' vulnerability as receivers of highly invasive medical procedures. Cultural and societal expectations related to parenting also add significant pressure on new mothers who want to demonstrate their maternal capacities lest they not experience judgment (this is discussed further in Chapter 3).

Sleep Disturbances

Sleep disturbances are strongly associated with PTSD, other trauma-related conditions, and anxiety disorders. Sleep difficulties in trauma survivors are connected to the changes in arousal and reactivity that trauma causes, although the exact biological mechanisms are complex. While sleep disturbances are an inherent part of the postpartum adjustment, sleep difficulties that don't improve in the postpartum year are associated with PPD (Lewis et al., 2018) and trauma (Swanson et al., 2014). ACOG (2012) mentions sleep disturbances as a possible non-acute symptom of IPV. Sleep disturbances are impossible to assess in the perinatal period with usual standards for sleep hygiene, making it challenging for perinatal clinicians to assess, especially in the context of trauma treatment. It is important to avoid both over-pathologizing and underestimating sleep issues for the perinatal mother. Her subjective sense of her sleep issues must be carefully assessed, including her previous relationship with sleep and sleep hygiene, and her current functioning. Caring for a newborn changes sleep patterns, especially for new mothers who breastfeed. But a new mother with a trauma history might assume her changes in sleep are normal parts of the postpartum phase if she had chronic untreated trauma-related sleep disturbances pre-pregnancy.

A study by Swanson et al. (2014) compared sleep issues in mothers with a history of childhood trauma. PTSD was associated with sleep problems. Mothers who had recovered from PTSD were more likely to have sleep issues than mothers exposed to childhood trauma who never developed PTSD. Mothers with persistent PTSD were at the highest risk for sleep problems. Sleep disturbances also increased thoughts of self-harm in postpartum women with depression (Sit et al., 2015). As with all symptoms of PMADs, a mother's developmental background for her sleep issues is crucial to assess.

Sleep protection is an extremely important factor for postpartum women's emotional state and requires extensive psychoeducation and often engagement of the social support system. Unrealistic expectations for a new mother's ability to provide constant infant care can contribute to a culture that normalizes severe sleep deprivation for mothers (the issue of unrealistic expectations for mothers will be addressed in Chapter 3). Furthermore, expectations for a new mother's ability to sleep when her baby is sleeping or when getting intermittent help with childcare can be unrealistic if her sleep issues are related to underlying traumatic stress or anxiety. The common message to new mothers that they should "sleep when the baby sleeps" can be insensitive and potentially harmful from a trauma-informed perspective. When exploring sleep issues and providing psychoeducation about the importance of sleep, clinicians must be careful not to make assumptions about a new mother's sleep abilities but should invite collaboratory exploration of potential ways to increase and protect her sleep. Many sleep issues will be related to underlying trauma-related hyperarousal and dysregulation that brings the mother to treatment. Sensory awareness skills (presented in Chapter 6) that facilitate the down-regulation of hyperarousal can be targeted towards sleep issues.

When assessing sleep disturbances in perinatal clients, it is important to explore and distinguish between difficulties falling asleep (sleep latency), sleep duration, night wakings (sleep disturbance), and subjective sleep quality. For all of these, it is also necessary to explore the relational contexts of how infant care activities, partner dynamics, and social support are impacting sleep. Other symptoms like negative thinking, hyperarousal, intrusive thoughts, or irritability must also be explored in relation to the specific sleep disturbances to get a sense of how they are triggered, maintained, and exacerbated. This contextual approach is necessary for biopsychosocial trauma treatment.

One client might present with problems falling and staying asleep due to rumination, intrusive thoughts, and hyperarousal, which could be related to high levels of trauma-related stress. Another client might present with little to no problems falling asleep, but with difficulties getting enough sleep due to hypervigilance about her baby making her feel unable to let others help with infant care. Some clients might present with issues of reducing their already limited sleep and rest time due to feeling compulsively drawn to childcare and practical activities, which could be related to underlying OCD symptoms. It is also important to explore environmental sleep hygiene factors like caffeine intake, sleeping arrangements, or electronic media use when assessing postpartum sleep issues (Lewis et al., 2018).

Flashbacks and Intrusive Thoughts

Re-experiencing symptoms often indicate high levels of trauma-related distress and distinguish PTSD from other disorders. Research has found that re-experiencing symptoms was the most accurate for identifying postpartum women who had traumatic births (Ayers et al., 2015b). However, clients can present with re-experiencing symptoms without meeting the criteria for PTSD (Diamond & Colaianni, 2022). Intrusive traumatic memories are characterized by marked increase in physiological distress and nervous system dysregulation and associated with the hyperarousal symptoms of PTSD (Stevens et al., 2021). Research suggests that the physical changes of pregnancy (specifically changes to the hypothalamic-pituitary-ovarian (HPO) axis and the hypothalamic-pituitary-adrenal (HPA) axis) increase PTSD symptoms making perinatal PTSD characterized by higher frequency and intensity of traumatic memories (Seng et al. 2005, Seng et al. 2010). Some mothers with high levels of anxiety and dysregulation might not recognize moments of distress as related to intrusive thoughts or flashbacks, especially if they have a history of dissociative symptoms too. In Beck's (2011) study, some mothers experienced that breastfeeding triggered flashbacks of the traumatic birth. Conversely, some mothers experienced breastfeeding as soothing and conducive to their recovery.

Intrusive thoughts related to traumatic memories should be distinguished from intrusive thoughts related to OCD, although they can overlap and co-occur. There is considerable comorbidity with around 19% of people with PTSD who also have OCD (Wadsworth et al., 2021). Furthermore, around half of those with an OCD diagnosis had one or more traumatic life events (Cromer et al., 2007). The perinatal period presents an increased risk for either onset or exacerbation of OCD (Fairbrother et al., 2021). Both intrusive thoughts and flashbacks of traumatic memories are ego-dystonic, meaning unwanted and experienced as foreign, which distinguishes them from psychotic delusions. Perinatal OCD is not associated with a risk of violent behavior (Fairbrother et al., 2021). Intrusive thoughts can, however, co-occur with suicidality, which is why intrusive thoughts never exclude assessment of suicidality. There is currently no data on whether intrusive thoughts about suicide or self-harm increase the risk of suicide; clinicians should assess for both suicidality and OCD (2020Mom, 2022).

Avoidance and Dissociation

For several forms of perinatal trauma, a woman's body and her baby can be trauma reminders or triggers and influence symptoms of avoidance (Ayers et al., 2016; Kendall-Tackett, 2017). For some mothers, intrusive thoughts about harming the baby are so disturbing that she will avoid holding her baby as a way to reduce the overwhelm. Traumatic birth can cause avoidance of follow-up medical care (Kendall-Tackett, 2017), but pre-pregnancy trauma history can also cause it. Avoidance of follow-up care is highly problematic as it can trigger a snowball effect of negative consequences: If a mother avoids her postpartum follow-up, her recovery might be impacted, and treatable medical issues might worsen or contribute to subsequent complications. Furthermore, if physical complications go unaddressed, they can contribute to emotional health issues, especially negative emotions related to the somatic aspects of postpartum adjustment and pain. This cascading effect can continue in a vicious cycle. It is crucial to acknowledge that a mother's avoidance of care is self-protective. In the case of insensitive, discriminatory, or abusive providers or care systems, clinicians must never pathologize a mother's avoidance behavior but acknowledge it as both understandable and wise of her to avoid further trauma. Avoidance can occur in the form of avoidance of external reminders like places or people, or avoidance of memories, thoughts, and feelings.

The unique sensations and body processes of pregnancy and postpartum are often overwhelming, especially for the first-time mother who has little to no reference to make sense of her sensations (this is elaborated in Chapter 6). This can exacerbate trauma symptoms. What makes the perinatal situation difficult, often impossible, is that the new mother cannot avoid her body, bodily processes, and her baby, which puts her a risk for dissociation as a reaction to the overwhelm. Dissociation is associated with high levels of trauma-related stress and should promptly elicit comprehensive assessment and clinical attention. It is a risk factor strongly associated with childbirth-related PTSD (Ayers et al., 2016).

Many triggering circumstances cannot be avoided. For example, a new mother with a baby in the NICU has to go back to the hospital. Or a mother who depends on practical help from family members who are reminders of childhood abuse. It is crucial to explore the interactions between avoidance behavior and symptoms of dissociation in the context of the mother's practical situation. Research has supported the recognition of a PTSD-dissociation subtype (Stein et al., 2013), which is associated with more lifetime trauma and childhood maltreatment. A study also demonstrated that pregnant women with PTSD-dissociation subtype had higher cortisol than pregnant women with non-dissociative PTSD, and a control group (Seng et al., 2018). Sensory awareness skills presented in Chapter 6 are important clinical tools for addressing dissociation.

Negative Mood or Cognitions

The maternal transition is existentially intense and elicits a wide range of every thinkable emotion, including negative ones. Trauma and depression are highly comorbid and overlap in symptomology, especially in relation to negative mood. Detachment or estrangement, which is a common symptom of PTSD and trauma related to dissociation, must be understood in the context of the new mother having experienced nothing less than "a seismic shift" in her identity due to the transition to motherhood (McCarty, 2020). The perinatal period is unique in that a woman's negative feelings are always experienced in the context of expecting or having had a baby, which adds another layer to them. Depressed thoughts and feelings in the perinatal period are associated with shame and guilt (Meeussen & Van Laar, 2018). A mother's negative feelings may also impact her feelings towards her baby or partner (Kendall-Tackett, 2017). Perinatal clinicians must therefore assess the layers of the negative mood and thoughts and the woman's reactions to having them. Common screening tools for depressed mood like the Patient Health Questionnaire or Beck's Depressive Inventory and even the perinatal-specific Edinburgh Postpartum Depression Scale do not assess for these layers of guilt, shame, or ambivalence that mothers experience.

It is important to consider negative moods or cognitions in the context of the perinatal woman's pain levels, as negative emotions interact with pain. A study by Goutaudier et al. (2012) demonstrated that negative emotions were significant predictors of the intensity of postpartum PTSS and that the combination of high levels of negative emotions with high levels of pain were even stronger predictors of PTSS. The entire perinatal transition can involve many forms of pain that are unfamiliar to expecting and new mothers, for example, childbirth recovery or muscle tension from breastfeeding positions. Pain issues can be overlooked and dismissed by both mothers and providers, especially if they are part of the non-pathological bodily processes of pregnancy and postpartum. Perinatal clinicians should not minimize pain in the perinatal period and model a low tolerance for pain from a Mental Health perspective by consistently referring to pain management care.

Hyperarousal and Reactivity

The perinatal transition can be understood as a profound expansion of the nervous system that involves significant neurological, hormonal, and autonomic nervous system changes (discussed in Chapter 2). Changes in arousal patterns are therefore inherent to the perinatal period and must be normalized as such. At the same time, it is important that clinicians don't minimize hyperarousal symptoms that are related to perinatal trauma or traumatic stress. Pregnant women seem to be particularly susceptible to hyperarousal symptoms of PTSD (Kornfield et al., 2018). Research has confirmed hyperarousal symptoms as a common phenomenon for perinatal women but found that they have poor specificity making them hard to assess and use for assessment of trauma (Ayers et al., 2015b). This is why it is important for clinicians to be sensitive and knowledgeable about dysregulation, as screening tools are no substitute for careful contextual assessment of a new mother's hyperarousal. Above all, perinatal clinicians must establish therapeutic safety in order to effectively explore and understand a mother's symptoms of hypervigilance (discussed in Chapters 4 and 5).

Clinicians must assess the developmental history of a mother's nervous system patterns. Hypervigilance related to the maternal transition might be more intense and may qualitatively differ from anything a woman has ever experienced while still resembling pre-pregnancy reactivity patterns. It is helpful to explore other times in a mother's life when she experienced significant changes in her nervous system to understand precipitating and perpetuating factors, especially life events that were stressful or traumatic. It also helps to assess how and where the hypervigilance is directed. It can be generalized, focused on the baby, the mother herself, her health or physical symptoms, issues related to the baby's feeding, in reaction to medical care, or towards other family members, and situations of feeling judged.

Beck's (2011) study on mothers who had traumatic births found that some women became hypervigilant about protecting their bodies as a reaction to the feeling of having been physically violated during delivery. Hypervigilance is often related to the baby, but it's important to note that this can be experienced as part of maternal ambivalence and therefore be complex. A mother may be intensely hypervigilant about protecting her baby while at the same time feeling resentment, alienation, fear, anger, or disinterest towards her baby. It is important to explore if her hypervigilance is waxing and waning in response to concrete triggers and stressors or if it is chronically high.

Anger, Rage, and Irritability

The term "postpartum rage" has gained awareness in both perinatal therapist communities and public discourse. However, the topic remains neglected by research and no robust data on prevalence exists (Ou et al., 2022). Anger and irritability are recognized as possible symptoms of depression and can also be part of the trauma symptom category of changes in arousal and reactivity patterns. Emerging research indicates that anger can be a vulnerability factor for PMAD onset (Bruno et al., 2018). From a nervous system perspective, anger is related to the survival response system, specifically the stage of mobilization of defenses in response to threats (Norton et al., 2011). The experience of threat is unique for the expecting or new mother who is undergoing an expansion of her protective instincts for both her baby and her own increased vulnerability. Perinatal anger and rage must be explored in this nervous system context of self-protective impulses. Other biological factors like lack of sleep and fatigue, which are common perinatal stressors, have been linked to postpartum anger and depression (Ou et al., 2022). It is important to consider the societal context of anger and rage. The severe racial and ethnic disparities and health inequities in maternity care make anger a healthy and understandable response to systemic injustices. The systemic issues of health inequities in Maternal Health can be understood with Smith and Freyd's (2014) concept of institutional betrayal trauma (Granner & Seng, 2021).

Suicidality

Suicidality is a leading cause of maternal mortality in the US after methods for data collection have been changed to recognize maternal suicide as pregnancy-related deaths (Sit et al., 2015; 2020Mom, 2022). Suicide is associated with severe depression and PTSD (ACOG, 2012). Suicidal ideation and thoughts in the perinatal period have been linked to PPD (Orsolini et al., 2016) and traumatic birth (Howard et al., 2011). However, the relationship between suicidal thoughts and suicide attempts in the perinatal period is not clear (Howard et al., 2011).

Risk factors for suicide in the perinatal period include not receiving Mental Health treatment, younger maternal age, unpartnered relationship status, unplanned pregnancy, non-Caucasian race, shorter illness duration, pre-existing, and/or current psychiatric diagnosis (Reid et al., 2022). Furthermore, a history of abuse increases the risk of suicidality in the perinatal period (2020Mom, 2022). Mental Health disorders like Major Depressive Disorder, Bipolar Disorder, and psychotic disorders present a higher risk of suicidality, also in the perinatal period (Orsolini et al., 2016). Lack of social support during the perinatal period is also strongly associated with suicidal behavior (2020Mom, 2022).

Suicidality in the perinatal period is clinically complex. Mothers with PPD can present with thoughts of self-harm without suicidal ideation; making it important that clinicians conduct a thorough safety assessment (Sit et al., 2015). Item 10 on the Edinburg Postnatal Depression Scale assesses thoughts of self-harm with the options for answers being "quite often", "sometimes", "hardly ever", and "never". Any response besides "never" should be followed up with assessment or referrals. It is important to note that while thoughts of self-harm are not synonymous with suicidal ideation, research has demonstrated that endorsement of "often" usually indicates significant suicidality and depression warranting referral for further assessment (Howard et al., 2011).

A Biopsychosocial Approach to Trauma-Informed Perinatal Care

Focusing on trauma in Perinatal Mental Health is not optional. Yet, despite growing amounts of research demonstrating the connections between trauma and PMADs, few models of perinatal care explicitly emphasize trauma-informed care (TIC) (Polmanteer et al., 2019; Seng & Taylor, 2015). Trauma-informed perinatal care is built on awareness of how past trauma can impact a woman's maternal transition, sensitivity to the risks of traumatization during the perinatal period, and active measures to prevent and mitigate traumatic stress reactions related to all aspects of the perinatal transition (Seng & Taylor, 2015). TIC recognizes the life-long impacts of trauma on biological, psychological, and social levels, and implements accommodations that limit or eliminate the influence of trauma (Elliott et al., 2005).

TIC requires providers to prioritize building supportive relationships with clients through empathy, respect, and validation (Polmanteer et al., 2019), which are already considered important factors for perinatal care (Davis et al., 2020). TIC is particularly important for mothers from diverse and marginalized groups who are disproportionately affected by trauma and are less likely to receive treatment (Polmanteer et al., 2019; Seng & Taylor, 2015). SAMHSA's (2014a) principles for TIC include safety, trustworthiness and transparency, peer support, collaboration and mutuality, empowerment, voice, and choice, and historical, cultural, racial, ethnic, gender, and diversity issues. These principles inform the model of *Somatic Maternal Healing* as shown in Table 0.1.

TABLE 0.1 Application of SAMHSA's Principles of Trauma-Informed Care in Somatic Maternal Healing

Principles for Trauma-Informed Care	Somatic Maternal Healing	Clinical Skills
Safety	No rushing the treatment process. Verbal and nonverbal acknowledgement of psychobiological aspects of trauma and stress: ♦ Nervous system psychoeducation ♦ Attunement: Therapist tracks own and client's nervous system	Coregulation and nonverbal communication, Chapter 5. Sensory awareness skills; slowing down, nervous system tracking, Chapter 6.
Trustworthiness and transparency	Psychoeducation about perinatal trauma and its systemic factors. Therapist is open about how they are conceptualizing client's situation and planning the treatment.	Psychoeducation on perinatal trauma and bottom-up treatment, Chapters 4 and 8. Trauma-responsive and empowering psychoeducation, Chapter 8.
Peer support	Focus on social and relational support in the therapeutic relationship and beyond. Needs for referrals to resources besides therapy continuously assessed and offered with special emphasis on anti-inflammatory and stress-reducing interventions.	Psychoeducation on biomedical aspects of PMADs and perinatal trauma, Chapter 2. Holistic treatment planning, Chapter 8.
Collaboration and mutuality	Focus on subjective experience of mother. Focus on coregulation as central to the therapeutic relationship.	Supporting assertion of embodied maternal subjectivity, Chapter 1. Coregulation, Chapter 5.
Empowerment, voice, and choice	Distinguishing between the societal institution of motherhood and its oppressive effects vs. mothering as diverse practices and expressions of the individual.	Feminist and empowered mothering, Chapter 3. Supporting maternal bodyfulness, Chapters 3 and 6.

(Cont.)

TABLE 0.1 (Cont.)

Principles for Trauma-Informed Care	Somatic Maternal Healing	Clinical Skills
	Focus on mother's assertion of her embodied subjectivity and ways she is resisting patriarchal motherhood.	
Historical, cultural, racial, ethnic, gender, and diversity issues	Acknowledgement of and transparency about the significant disparities in perinatal care and systemic and societal issues contributing to client's situation. Focus on client's subjective experience and valuing it. Inviting client's feedback and wishes for treatment. Respecting client's belief system and cultural practices and acknowledging client's use of them for healing.	Supporting assertion of embodied maternal subjectivity, Chapter 1. Supporting maternal bodyfulness, Chapters 3 and 6.

References

2020Mom. (2022, October). *Maternal suicide in the U.S. Opportunities for improved data collection and health care system change (Issue Brief)*. 2020Mom.org. Retrieved from https://www.2020mom.org/maternal-suicide

Alcorn, K.L., O'Donovan, A., Patrick, J.C., Creedy, D., & Devilly, G.J. (2010). A prospective longitudinal study of the prevalence of post-traumatic stress disorder resulting from childbirth events. *Psychological Medicine, 40*(11), 1849–1859. 10.1017/S0033291709992224

Alhusen, J.L., Ray, E., Sharps, P., & Bullock, L. (2015). Intimate partner violence during pregnancy: Maternal and neonatal outcomes. *Journal of Women's Health, 24*(1), 100–106. 10.1089/jwh.2014.4872

American College of Obstetricians and Gynecologists Committee Opinion No. 518: Intimate partner violence. (2012). *Obstetrics and Gynecology, 119*(2 Pt 1), 412–417. 10.1097/AOG.0b013e318249ff74

American Psychiatric Association. (2022). *Diagnostic and statistical manual of mental disorders* (5th ed., text rev.). 10.1176/appi.books.9780890425787

Ayers, S. (2017). Birth trauma and post-traumatic stress disorder: The importance of risk and resilience. *Journal of Reproductive and Infant Psychology*, 35(5), 427–430. 10.1080/02646838.2017.1386874

Ayers, S., Bond, R., Bertullies, S., & Wijma, K. (2016). The aetiology of post-traumatic stress following childbirth: A meta-analysis and theoretical framework. *Psychological Medicine*, 46(6), 1121–1134. 10.1017/S0033291715002706

Ayers, S., Eagle, A., & Waring, H. (2006). The effects of childbirth-related post-traumatic stress disorder on women and their relationships: A qualitative study. *Psychological Health and Medicine*, 11(4), 389–398. 10.1080/13548500600708409

Ayers, S., McKenzie-McHarg, K., & Slade, P. (2015a). Post-traumatic stress disorder after birth. *Journal of Reproductive and Infant Psychology*, 33(3), 215–218. 10.1080/02646838.2015.1030250

Ayers, S., Wright, D.B., & Ford, E. (2015b). Traumatic birth and hyperarousal symptoms: Are they normal or pathological? *Journal of Reproductive and Infant Psychology, Special Issue*, 33(3), 282–293.

Bajaj, M.A., Salimgaraev, R., Zhaunova, L., & Payne, J.L. (2022). Rates of self-reported postpartum depressive symptoms in the United States before and after the start of the COVID-19 pandemic. *Journal of Psychiatric Research*, 151, 108–112. 10.1016/j.jpsychires.2022.04.011

Beck, C.T. (2004). Birth trauma: In the eye of the beholder. *Nursing Research*, 53, 28–35. 10.1097/00006199-200401000-00005

Beck, C.T. (2011). A metaethnography of traumatic childbirth and its aftermath: Amplifying causal looping. *Qualitative Health Research*, 21(3), 301–311. 10.1177/1049732310390698

Beck, C.T., Driscoll, J.W., & Watson, S. (2013). *Traumatic childbirth*. Routledge. 10.4324/9780203766699

Becker-Sadzio, J., Gundel, F., Kroczek, A., Wekenmann, S., Rapp, A., Fallgatter, A.J., & Deppermann, S. (2020). Trauma exposure therapy in a pregnant woman suffering from complex post-traumatic stress disorder after childhood sexual abuse: Risk or benefit? *European Journal of Psychotraumatology*, 11(1), 1697581. 10.1080/20008198.2019.1697581

Bonde, J.P.E., Jensen, J.H., Smid, G.E., Flachs, E.M., Elklit, A., Mors, O., & Videbech, P. (2022). Time course of symptoms in posttraumatic stress disorder with delayed expression: A systematic review. *Acta Psychiatrica Scandinavica, 145*(2), 116–131. 10.1111/acps.13372

Braveman, P., Dominguez, T.P., Burke, W., Dolan, S.M., Stevenson, D.K., Jackson, F.M., Collins, J.W., Jr, Driscoll, D.A., Haley, T., Acker, J., Shaw, G.M., McCabe, E.R.B., Hay, W.W., Jr, Thornburg, K., Acevedo-Garcia, D., Cordero, J.F., Wise, P.H., Legaz, G., Rashied-Henry, K., Frost, J., ...Waddell, L. (2021). Explaining the black-white disparity in preterm birth: A consensus statement from a multi-disciplinary scientific work group convened by the March of Dimes. *Frontiers in Reproductive Health, 3*, 684207. 10.3389/frph.2021.684207

Bruno, A., Laganà, A.S., Leonardi, V., Greco, D., Merlino, M., Vitale, S.G., Triolo, O., Zoccali, R.A., & Muscatello, M.R.A. (2018). Inside-out: The role of anger experience and expression in the development of postpartum mood disorders. *The Journal of Maternal-Fetal & Neonatal Medicine, 31*(22), 3033–3038. 10.1080/14767058.2017.1362554

Chen, Q., Li, W., Xiong, J., & Zheng, X. (2022). Prevalence and risk factors associated with postpartum depression during the COVID-19 pandemic: A literature review and meta-analysis. *International Journal of Environmental Research and Public Health, 19*(4), 2219. 10.3390/ijerph19042219

Choi, K.W., & Sikkema, K.J. (2016). Childhood maltreatment and perinatal mood and anxiety disorders: A systematic review. *Trauma, Violence & Abuse, 17*(5), 427–453. 10.1177/1524838015584369

Cook, N., Ayers, S., & Horsch, A. (2018). Maternal posttraumatic stress disorder during the perinatal period and child outcomes: A systematic review. *Journal of Affective Disorders, 225*, 18–31. 10.1016/j.jad.2017.07.045

Crawley, R., Lomax, S., & Ayers, S. (2013). Recovering from stillbirth: The effects of making and sharing memories on Maternal Mental Health. *Journal of Reproductive and Infant Psychology, 31*, 195–207.

Creedy, D.K., Shochet, I.M., & Horsfall, J. (2000). Childbirth and the development of acute trauma symptoms: Incidence and contributing factors. *Birth (Berkeley, Calif.), 27*(2), 104–111. 10.1046/j.1523-536x.2000.00104.x

Cromer, K.R., Schmidt, N.B., & Murphy, D.L. (2007). An investigation of traumatic life events and obsessive-compulsive disorder. *Behaviour Research and Therapy, 45,* 1683–1691. 10.1016/j.brat.2006.08.018.

Davis, W., McCue, K., Papierniak, B., Raines, C., & Simanis, L. (2020). Emotional and practical needs in postpartum women. The role of family and friend support and social network. In R.M. Quatraro, & P. Grusse (Eds.), *Handbook of perinatal clinical psychology. From theory to practice* (pp. 189–199). Routledge. 10.4324/9780429351990

Delicate, A., Ayers, S., & McMullen, S. (2020). Health care practitioners' views of the support women, partners, and the couple relationship require for birth trauma: Current practice and potential improvements. *Primary Health Care Research & Development, 21,* e40. 10.1017/S1463423620000407

Diamond, R.M., & Colaianni, A. (2022). The impact of perinatal healthcare changes on birth trauma during COVID-19. *Women and Birth: Journal of the Australian College of Midwives, 35*(5), 503–510. 10.1016/j.wombi.2021.12.003

Elliott, D.E., Bjelajac, P., Fallot, R.D., Markoff, L.S., & Reed, R.G. (2005). Trauma-informed or trauma-denied: Principles and implementation of trauma-informed services for women. *Journal of Community Psychology, 33*(4), 461–477. 10.1002/jcop.20063

Ely, D.M., & Driscoll, A.K. (2022). Infant mortality in the United States, 2020: Data from the period linked birth/infant death file. *National Vital Statistics Reports: From the Centers for Disease Control and Prevention, National Center for Health Statistics, National Vital Statistics System, 71*(5), 1–18. Retrieved from https://www.cdc.gov/nchs/data/nvsr/nvsr71/nvsr71-05.pdf

Fairbrother, N., Collardeau, F., Albert, A.Y.K., Challacombe, F.L., Thordarson, D.S., Woody, S.R., & Janssen, P.A. (2021). High prevalence and incidence of Obsessive-Compulsive Disorder among women across pregnancy and the postpartum. *The Journal of Clinical Psychiatry, 82*(2), 20m13398. 10.4088/JCP.20m13398

Fisher, J., Acton, C., & Rowe, H. (2018). Mental health problems among childbearing women: Historical perspectives and social determinants. In M. Muzik, & K.L. Rosenblum (Eds.), *Motherhood in the face of trauma: Pathways towards healing and growth* (pp. 3–20). Springer. 10.1007/978-3-319-65724-0

Ford, E., & Ayers, S. (2011). Support during birth interacts with trauma history and birth intervention to predict postnatal post-traumatic stress symptoms. *Psychology & Health, 26*, 1553–1570. 10.1080/08870446.2010.533770

Franke, H. (2014). Toxic stress: Effects, prevention, and treatment. *Children, 1*(3), 390–402. 10.3390/children1030390

Giannandrea, A.M., Cerulli, C., Anson, E., & Chaudron, L.H. (2013). Increased risk for postpartum psychiatric disorders among women with past pregnancy loss. *Journal of Women's Health, 22*(9), 760–768. 10.1089/jwh.2012.4011

Giurgescu, C., & Misra, D.P. (2018). Psychosocial factors and preterm birth among black mothers and fathers. *MCN. The American Journal of Maternal Child Nursing, 43*(5), 245–251. 10.1097/NMC.0000000000000458

Gold, K.J., Leon, I., Boggs, M.E., & Sen, A. (2016). Depression and post-traumatic stress symptoms after perinatal loss in a population-based sample. *Journal of Women's Health (2002), 25*(3), 263–269. 10.1089/jwh.2015.5284

Goutaudier, N., Séjourné, N., Rousset, C., Lami, C., & Chabrol, H. (2012). Negative emotions, childbirth pain, perinatal dissociation, and self-efficacy as predictors of postpartum posttraumatic stress symptoms. *Journal of Reproductive and Infant Psychology, 30*(4), 352–362, 10.1080/02646838.2012.738415

Granner, J.R., & Seng, J.S. (2021). Using theories of posttraumatic stress to inform perinatal care clinician responses to trauma reactions. *Journal of Midwifery & Women's Health, 66*(5), 567–578. 10.1111/jmwh.13287

Greenfield, M., Jomeen, J., & Glover, L. (2016). What is traumatic birth? A concept analysis and literature review. *British Journal of Midwifery, 24*, 254–267. 10.12968/bjom.2016.24.4.254

Grekin, R., Brock, R.L., & O'Hara, M.W. (2017). The effects of trauma on perinatal depression: Examining trajectories of depression from pregnancy through 24 months postpartum in an at-risk population. *Journal of Affective Disorders, 218*, 269–276. 10.1016/j.jad.2017.04.051

Grisbrook, M.A., & Letourneau, N. (2021). Improving maternal post-partum mental health screening guidelines requires assessment of post-traumatic stress disorder. *Canadian Journal of Public Health, 112*(2), 240–243. 10.17269/s41997-020-00373-8

Guidi, J., Lucente, M., Sonino, N., & Fava, G.A. (2021). Allostatic load and its impact on health: A systematic review. *Psychotherapy and Psychosomatics*, *90*(1), 11–27. 10.1159/000510696

Guintivano, J., Manuck, T., & Meltzer-Brody, S. (2018). Predictors of Postpartum Depression: A comprehensive review of the last decade of evidence. *Clinical Obstetrics and Gynecology*, *61*(3), 591–603. 10.1097/GRF.0000000000000368

Horsch, A., Jacobs, I., & McKenzie-McHarg, K. (2015). Cognitive predictors and risk factors of maternal posttraumatic stress disorder following stillbirth: A longitudinal study. *Journal of Reproductive Infant Psychology*, *33*, E22–E23. 10.1002/jts.21997

Howard, L.M., Flach, C., Mehay, A., Sharp, D., & Tylee, A. (2011). The prevalence of suicidal ideation identified by the Edinburgh Postnatal Depression Scale in postpartum women in primary care: Findings from the RESPOND trial. *BMC Pregnancy and Childbirth*, *11*, 57. 10.1186/1471-2393-11-57

Huffhines, L., Coe, J.L., Busuito, A., Seifer, R., & Parade, S.H. (2022). Understanding links between maternal perinatal posttraumatic stress symptoms and infant socioemotional and physical health. *Infant Mental Health Journal*, *43*, 474–492. 10.1002/imhj.21985

James, L., Brody, D., & Hamilton, Z. (2013). Risk factors for domestic violence during pregnancy: A meta-analytic review. *Violence and Victims*, *28*(3), 359–380. 10.1891/0886-6708.vv-d-12-00034

Jokić, B., Purić, D., Grassmann, H., Walling, C.G., Nix, E.J., Porges, S.W., & Kolacz, J. (2022). Association of childhood maltreatment with adult body awareness and autonomic reactivity: The moderating effect of practicing body psychotherapy. *Psychotherapy (Chicago, Ill.)*, 10.1037/pst0000463. Advance online publication. 10.1037/pst0000463

Kendall-Tackett, K.A. (2017). *Depression in new mothers. Causes, consequences, and treatment alternatives* (3rd ed.). Routledge.

Kornfield, S.L., Hantsoo, L., & Epperson, C.N. (2018). What does sex have to do with it? The role of sex as a biological variable in the development of posttraumatic stress disorder. *Current Psychiatry Reports*, *20*(6), 39. 10.1007/s11920-018-0907-x

Kornfield, S.L., Johnson, R.L., Hantsoo, L.V., Kaminsky, R.B., Waller, R., Sammel, M., & Epperson, C.N. (2022). Engagement in and benefits of a short-term, brief psychotherapy intervention for PTSD during pregnancy. *Frontiers in Psychiatry*, *13*, 882429. 10.3389/fpsyt.2022.882429

Kuhfuß, M., Maldei, T., Hetmanek, A., & Baumann, N. (2021). Somatic experiencing – effectiveness and key factors of a body-oriented trauma therapy: A scoping literature review. *European Journal of Psychotraumatology, 12*, 1929023. 10.1080/20008198.2021.1929023

Levine, P.A. (2010). *In an unspoken voice. How the body releases trauma and restores goodness.* North Atlantic Books.

Lewis, B.A., Gjerdingen, D., Schuver, K., Avery, M., & Marcus, B.H. (2018). The effect of sleep pattern changes on postpartum depressive symptoms. *BMC Women's Health, 18*(1), 12. 10.1186/s12905-017-0496-6

MacDorman, M.F., & Gregory, E.C. (2015). Fetal and perinatal mortality: United States, 2013. *National Vital Statistics Reports: From the Centers for Disease Control and Prevention, National Center for Health Statistics, National Vital Statistics System, 64*(8), 1–24. Retrieved from https://www.cdc.gov/nchs/data/nvsr/nvsr64/nvsr64_08.pdf

Martínez-Vazquez, S., Rodríguez-Almagro, J., Hernández-Martínez, A., Delgado-Rodríguez, M., & Martínez-Galiano, J.M. (2021). Long-term high risk of postpartum post-traumatic stress disorder (PTSD) and associated factors. *Journal of Clinical Medicine, 10*(3), 488. 10.3390/jcm10030488

Maté, G. (2010). *In the realm of the hungry ghosts: Close encounters with addiction.* North Atlantic Books.

Matthews, K., Morgan, I., Davis, K., Estriplet, T., Perez, S., & Crear-Perry, J.A. (2021). Pathways to equitable and antiracist maternal mental health care: Insights from black women stakeholders. *Health Affairs (Project Hope), 40*(10), 1597–1604. 10.1377/hlthaff.2021.00808

Mayopoulos, G.A., Ein-Dor, T., Li, K.G., Chan, S.J., & Dekel, S. (2021). COVID-19 positivity associated with traumatic stress response to childbirth and no visitors and infant separation in the hospital. *Scientific Reports, 11*(1), 13535. 10.1038/s41598-021-92985-4

McCarthy, J. (2020). The corporeal dimensions of motherhood. In C. Arnold-Baker (Ed.), *The existential crisis of motherhood* (pp. 37–55). Palgrave Macmillan.

McEwen, B.S., & Stellar, E. (1993). Stress and the individual. Mechanisms leading to disease. *Archives of Internal Medicine, 153*(18), 2093–2101. 10.1001/archinte.1993.00410180039004

Meeussen, L., & Van Laar, C. (2018). Feeling pressure to be a perfect mother relates to parental burnout and career ambitions. *Frontiers in Psychology, 9*, 2113. 10.3389/fpsyg.2018.02113

Minckas, N., Medvedev, M.M., Adejuyigbe, E.A., Brotherton, H., Chellani, H., Estifanos, A.S., Ezeaka, C., Gobezayehu, A.G., Irimu, G., Kawaza, K., Kumar, V., Massawe, A., Mazumder, S., Mambule, I., Medhanyie, A.A., Molyneux, E.M., Newton, S., Salim, N., Tadele, H., Tann, C.J., …COVID-19 Small and Sick Newborn Care Collaborative Group (2021). Preterm care during the COVID-19 pandemic: A comparative risk analysis of neonatal deaths averted by kangaroo mother care versus mortality due to SARS-CoV-2 infection. *EClinicalMedicine, 33*, 100733. 10.1016/j.eclinm.2021.100733

Morelen, D., Rosenblum, K.L., & Muzik, M. (2018). Childhood maltreatment and motherhood: Implications for maternal well-being and mothering. In M. Muzik, & K.L. Rosenblum (Eds.), *Motherhood in the face of trauma. Pathways towards healing and growth* (pp. 23–37). Springer. 10.1007/978-3-319-65724-0_2

Mylle, J., & Maes, M. (2004). Partial posttraumatic stress disorder revisited. *Journal of Affective Disorders, 78*(1), 37–48. 10.1016/s0165-0327(02)00218-5

Nillni, Y.I., Mehralizade, A., Mayer, L., & Milanovic, S. (2018). Treatment of depression, anxiety, and trauma-related disorders during the perinatal period: A systematic review. *Clinical Psychology Review, 66*, 136–148. 10.1016/j.cpr.2018.06.004

Norton, B., Ferriegel, M., & Norton, C. (2011). Somatic expressions of trauma in experiential play therapy. *International Journal of Play Therapy, 20*(3), 138–152. 10.1037/a0024349

O'Hara, M.W., & Wisner, K.L. (2014). Perinatal mental illness: Definition, description, and aetiology. *Best Practice & Research Clinical Obstetrics & Gynaecology, 28*(1), 3–12. 10.1016/j.bpobgyn.2013.09.002

Olff, M. (2017). Sex and gender differences in post-traumatic stress disorder: An update. *European Journal of Psychotraumatology, 8*(4). 10.1080/20008198.2017.1351204

Orsolini, L., Valchera, A., Vecchiotti, R., Tomasetti, C., Iasevoli, F., Fornaro, M., De Berardis, D., Perna, G., Pompili, M., & Bellantuono, C. (2016). Suicide during perinatal period: Epidemiology, risk factors, and clinical correlates. *Frontiers in Psychiatry, 7*, 138. 10.3389/fpsyt.2016.00138

Ou, C.H., Hall, W.A., Rodney, P., & Stremler, R. (2022). Correlates of Canadian mothers' anger during the postpartum period: A cross-sectional survey. *BMC Pregnancy and Childbirth, 22*(1), 163. 10.1186/s12884-022-04479-4

Padin, A.C., Stevens, N.R., Che, M.L., Erondu, I.N., Perera, M.J., & Shalowitz, M.U. (2022). Screening for PTSD during pregnancy: A missed opportunity. *BMC Pregnancy and Childbirth*, *22*(1), 487. 10.1186/s12884-022-04797-7

Payne, Peter, Levine, Peter A., & Crane-Godreau, Mardi A. (2015). Somatic experiencing: using interoception and proprioception as core elements of trauma therapy. *Frontiers in Psychology*, 6, 93. https://doi.org/10.3389/fpsyg.2015.00093

Perizzolo Pointet, V.C., Moser, D.A., Suardi, F., Rothenberg, M., Serpa, S.R., Schechter, D.S. (2018). Maternal trauma and related psychopathology: Consequences to parental brain functioning associated with caregiving. In M. Muzik, & K.L. Rosenblum (Eds.), *Motherhood in the face of trauma. Pathways towards healing and growth* (pp. 99–112). Springer. 10.1007/978-3-319-65724-0_7

Polmanteer, R.S.R., Keefe, R.H., & Brownstein-Evans, C. (2019). Trauma-informed care with women diagnosed with postpartum depression: A conceptual framework. *Social Work in Health Care*, *58*(2), 220–235. 10.1080/00981389.2018.1535464

Porges, S.W. (2022). Polyvagal theory: A science of safety. *Frontiers in Integrative Neuroscience*, *16*, 871227. 10.3389/fnint.2022.871227

Rao, S.P.N., Minckas, N., Medvedev, M.M., Gathara, D., Y N, P., Seifu Estifanos, A., Silitonga, A.C., Jadaun, A.S., Adejuyigbe, E.A., Brotherton, H., Arya, S., Gera, R., Ezeaka, C.V., Gai, A., Gobezayehu, A.G., Dube, Q., Kumar, A., Naburi, H., Chiume, M., Tumukunde, V., ...COVID-19 Small and Sick Newborn Care Collaborative Group (2021). Small and sick newborn care during the COVID-19 pandemic: Global survey and thematic analysis of healthcare providers' voices and experiences. *BMJ Global Health*, *6*(3), e004347. 10.1136/bmjgh-2020-004347

Reid, H.E., Pratt, D., Edge, D., & Wittkowski, A. (2022). Maternal suicide ideation and behaviour during pregnancy and the first postpartum year: A systematic review of psychological and psychosocial risk factors. *Frontiers in Psychiatry*, *13*, 765118. 10.3389/fpsyt.2022.765118

Sachdeva, J., Nagle Yang, S., Gopalan, P., Worley, L.L.M., Mittal, L., Shirvani, N., Spada, M., Albertini, E., Shenai, N., Moore Simas, T.A., & Byatt, N. (2022). Trauma informed care in the obstetric setting and role of the perinatal psychiatrist: A comprehensive review of the literature. *Journal of the Academy of Consultation-Liaison Psychiatry, 63*(5), 485–496. 10.1016/j.jaclp.2022.04.005

Sanjuan, P.M., Fokas, K., Tonigan, J.S., Henry, M.C., Christian, K., Rodriguez, A., Larsen, J., Yonke, N., & Leeman, L. (2021). Prenatal maternal posttraumatic stress disorder as a risk factor for adverse birth weight and gestational age outcomes: A systematic review and meta-analysis. *Journal of Affective Disorders, 295*, 530–540. 10.1016/j.jad.2021.08.079

Sareen, J. (2014). Posttraumatic stress disorder in adults: Impact, comorbidity, risk factors, and treatment. *The Canadian Journal of Psychiatry, 59*(9), 460–467. 10.1177/070674371405900902

Schore, A.N. (2013). Relational trauma, brain development, and dissociation. In J.D. Ford, & C.A. Courtois (Eds.), *Treating traumatic stress disorders in children and adolescents. Scientific foundations and therapeutic models* (pp. 3–23). Guilford Press.

Schore, A.N. (2021). The interpersonal neurobiology of intersubjectivity. *Frontiers in Psychology, 12*, 648616. 10.3389/fpsyg.2021.648616

Séjourné, N., & Goutaudier, N. (2020). Miscarriage and pregnancy loss. In R.M. Quatraro, & P. Grussu (Eds.), *Handbook of perinatal clinical psychology. From theory to practice* (pp. 103–131). Routledge. 10.4324/9780429351990

Seng, J., & Taylor, J. (Eds.). (2015). *Trauma informed care and the perinatal period*. Dunedin Academic Press.

Seng, J.S., Kohn-Wood, L.P., McPherson, M.D., & Sperlich, M. (2011). Disparity in posttraumatic stress disorder diagnosis among African American pregnant women. *Archives of Women's Mental Health, 14*(4), 295–306. 10.1007/s00737-011-0218-2

Seng, J.S., Li, Y., Yang, J.J., King, A.P., Kane Low, L.M., Sperlich, M., Rowe, H., Lee, H., Muzik, M., Ford, J.D., & Liberzon, I. (2018). Gestational and postnatal cortisol profiles of women with posttraumatic stress disorder and the dissociative subtype. *Journal of Obstetric, Gynecologic, and Neonatal Nursing, 47*(1), 12–22. 10.1016/j.jogn.2017.10.008

Seng, J.S., Low, L.K., Ben-Ami, D., & Liberzon, I. (2005). Cortisol level and perinatal outcome in pregnant women with posttraumatic stress disorder: A pilot study. *Journal of Midwifery & Women's Health, 50*(5), 392–398. 10.1016/j.jmwh.2005.04.024

Seng, J.S., Low, L.K., Sperlich, M., Ronis, D.L., & Liberzon, I. (2009). Prevalence, trauma history, and risk for posttraumatic stress disorder among nulliparous women in maternity care. *Obstetrics and Gynecology, 114*(4), 839–847. 10.1097/AOG.0b013e3181b8f8a2

Seng, J.S., Rauch, S.A., Resnick, H., Reed, C.D., King, A., Low, L.K., McPherson, M., Muzik, M., Abelson, J., & Liberzon, I. (2010). Exploring posttraumatic stress disorder symptom profile among pregnant women. *Journal of Psychosomatic Obstetrics and Gynaecology, 31*(3), 176–187. 10.3109/0167482X.2010.486453

Sit, D., Luther, J., Buysse, D., Dills, J.L., Eng, H., Okun, M., Wisniewski, S., & Wisner, K.L. (2015). Suicidal ideation in depressed postpartum women: Associations with childhood trauma, sleep disturbance, and anxiety. *Journal of Psychiatric Research, 66-67*, 95–104. 10.1016/j.jpsychires.2015.04.021

Smith, C.P., & Freyd, J.J. (2014). Institutional betrayal. *American Psychologist, 69*, 575–587. 10.1037/a0037564

Souch, A.J., Jones, I.R., Shelton, K.H.M., & Waters, C.S. (2022). Maternal childhood maltreatment and perinatal outcomes: A systematic review. *Journal of Affective Disorders, 302*, 139–159. 10.1016/j.jad.2022.01.062

Stein, D.J., Koenen, K.C., Friedman, M.J., Hill, E., McLaughlin, K.A., Petukhova, M., Ruscio, A.M., Shahly, V., Spiegel, D., Borges, G., Bunting, B., Caldas-de-Almeida, J.M., de Girolamo, G., Demyttenaere, K., Florescu, S., Haro, J.M., Karam, E.G., Kovess-Masfety, V., Lee, S., Matschinger, H., ... Kessler, R.C. (2013). Dissociation in posttraumatic stress disorder: Evidence from the world mental health surveys. *Biological Psychiatry, 73*(4), 302–312. 10.1016/j.biopsych.2012.08.022

Stevens, N.R., Miller, M.L., Puetz, A.K., Padin, A.C., Adams, N., & Meyer, D.J. (2021). Psychological intervention and treatment for posttraumatic stress disorder during pregnancy: A systematic review and call to action. *Journal of Traumatic Stress, 34*(3), 575–585. 10.1002/jts.22641

Substance Abuse and Mental Health Services Administration. (2014a). *SAMHSA's concept of trauma and guidance for a trauma-informed approach.* HHS Publication No. (SMA) 14–4884. Retrieved from https://ncsacw.acf.hhs.gov/userfiles/files/SAMHSA_Trauma.pdf

Substance Abuse and Mental Health Services Administration. (2014b). *Trauma-informed care in behavioral health services. Treatment improvement protocol (TIP)* Series 57. HHS Publication No. (SMA) 13–4801. Retrieved from https://www.ncbi.nlm.nih.gov/books/NBK207201/

Swanson, L.M., Hamilton, L., & Muzik, M. (2014). The role of childhood trauma and PTSD in postpartum sleep disturbance. *Journal of Traumatic Stress, 27*(6), 689–694. 10.1002/jts.21965

Tjaden, P.G., & Thoennes, N. (2000). *Full report of the prevalence, incidence, and consequences of violence against women. National Violence Against Women Survey.* National Institute of Justice (U.S.), Centers for Disease Control and Prevention (U.S.), National Center for Injury Prevention and Control (U.S.), NIJ special report. Retrieved from https://stacks.cdc.gov/view/cdc/21948

van de Kamp, M.M., Scheffers, M., Hatzmann, J., Emck, C., Cuijpers, P., & Beek, P.J. (2019). Body- and movement-oriented interventions for posttraumatic stress disorder: A systematic review and meta-analysis. *Journal of Traumatic Stress, 32*(6), 967–976. 10.1002/jts.22465

van der Kolk, B. (2015). *The body keeps the score: Brain, mind, and body in the healing of trauma.* Penguin Publishing.

Venta, A., Bick, J., & Bechelli, J. (2021). COVID-19 threatens maternal mental health and infant development: Possible paths from stress and isolation to adverse outcomes and a call for research and practice. *Child Psychiatry & Human Development, 52,* 200–204.

Verrault, N., DaCosta, D., & Marchand, A. (2012). PTSD following childbirth: A prospective study of incidence and risk factors in Canadian women. *Journal of Psychosomatic Research, 73,* 257–263.

Vignato, J., Georges, J.M., Bush, R.A., & Connelly, C.D. (2017). Post-traumatic stress disorder in the perinatal period: A concept analysis. *Journal of Clinical Nursing, 26*(23-24), 3859–3868. 10.1111/jocn.13800

Wadsworth, L.P., Van Kirk, N., August, M., Kelly, J.M., Jackson, F., Nelson, J., & Luehrs, R. (2021). *Understanding the overlap between OCD and trauma: Development of the OCD trauma timeline interview (OTTI) for clinical settings. Current psychology (New Brunswick, N.J.),* 1–11. Advance online publication. 10.1007/s12144-021-02118-3

Waller, R., Kornfield, S.L., White, L.K., Chaiyachati, B.H., Barzilay, R., Njoroge, W., Parish-Morris, J., Duncan, A., Himes, M.M., Rodriguez, Y., Seidlitz, J., Riis, V., Burris, H.H., Gur, R.E., & Elovitz, M.A. (2022). Clinician-reported childbirth outcomes, patient-reported childbirth trauma, and risk for postpartum depression. *Archives of Women's Mental Health 25,* 985–999. 10.1007/s00737-022-01263-3

Westby, C.L., Erlandsen, A.R., Nilsen, S.A., Visted, E., & Thimm, J.C. (2021). Depression, anxiety, PTSD, and OCD after stillbirth: A systematic review. *BMC Pregnancy and Childbirth, 21*(1), 782. 10.1186/s12884-021-04254-x

White, R.S., & Aaronson, J.A. (2022). Obstetric and perinatal racial and ethnic disparities. *Current Opinion in Anaesthesiology, 35*(3), 260–266. 10.1097/ACO.0000000000001133

World Health Organization. (2021). New research highlights risks of separating newborns from mothers during COVID-19 pandemic. Retrieved from: https://www.who.int/news/item/16-03-2021-new-research-highlights-risks-of-separating-newborns-frommothers-during-covid-19-pandemic

Yonkers, K.A., Smith, M.V., Forray, A., Epperson, C.N., Costello, D., & Lin, H. (2014). Pregnant women with post-traumatic stress disorder and risk of preterm birth. *JAMA Psychiatry, 71*, 897–904. 10.1001/jamapsychiatry.2014.558

1

The Question of Embodied Maternal Subjectivity

How Feminist Psychoanalysis Informs Clinical Work with Mothers

From Developmental Tasks of Maternal Identity Formation to Embodied Relational Subjectivity

When we look to psychoanalytic theory for insights into motherhood, we find both useful concepts and epistemological issues. The earlier generations of classic analytic writers began the first explorations by focusing on the developmental tasks of motherhood and maternal identity formation, starting with Freud's (1932) reflections on the connections between a woman's relationship with her own mother and her psychological adjustment to motherhood. Four main themes can be identified in the classic literature: Acceptance of the pregnancy and incorporation of the fetus (Bibring et al., 1961; Deutsch, 1945), recognition of the baby as a separate object (Bibring, 1959; Bibring et al., 1961; Pines, 1978), activation of the relationship with the woman's own mother and its possibility for resolving early conflicts (Deutsch, 1945; Freud, 1932, 1933; Mahler et al., 1975; Pines, 1982), and the bifurcated identification with the fetus and the woman's own mother (Bibring et al., 1961; Deutsch, 1945; Pines, 1978). A fifth transitional theme of the role and function of the body in the maternal transition is unique in that it has only been addressed by a few relatively unknown writers (Furman, 1982; Pines, 1978, 1994), and it is a key precursor for later contemporary developments. Furman and Pines explored the role of the body not only from the perspective of how the maternal body impacts the mother-infant relationship like the focus of Klein's thinking, but specifically from the perspective of having and being a maternal body and the psychological functions related to maternal embodiment. From this pioneering work, psychoanalytic thinking developed focusing on exploring the embodied aspects of maternal subjectivity and their implications for theory (Stone, 2014) and practice (Balsam, 2012; Orbach, 2006, 2009), and the issues with the absence of recognition of maternal subjectivity (Benjamin, 1995). As psychoanalysis evolved towards the intersubjective relational model, analytic thinking on motherhood also evolved to focus on the embodied relational subjectivity of mothers. However, these developments have been primarily theoretical.

Clinically focused psychodynamic approaches to Maternal Mental Health do exist but are few in number and do not constitute feminist psychoanalytic frameworks that address the issues of maternal embodied relational subjectivity. Menken (2008) has described a psychodynamic approach to the treatment of Postpartum Depression (PD) that focuses on maternal identity development from an attachment history perspective, aligned with the conceptualization of motherhood as a set of developmental tasks in classic analytic literature. From an object-relations perspective, Blum (2007) identified principal emotional conflicts of PD to be about dependency, anger, and the relationship to one's own mother, and discussed ways to address these as they come up in the transference. Kleiman (2017) developed an approach based on Winnicott's concept of holding as a set of directive techniques for immediate rapport-building and a clinical attitude of holding adapted to the unique needs of the perinatal client. While all valuable, none of these clinical approaches address the issues surrounding maternal embodied subjectivity and the role of trauma in the maternal transition. Contemporary psychoanalytic thinking about motherhood is primarily theory developed from the feminist engagement of the epistemological questions of maternal subjectivity and embodiment that were not adequately addressed in the classic literature. The main epistemological question here is the "problem" of maternal subjectivity which is deeply intertwined with the "problem" of maternal embodiment. This chapter will demonstrate how these two theoretical problems inform clinical work and how a deeper excavation of feminist psychoanalytic theory is crucial for trauma-informed (and therefore body-focused) therapy with mothers.

The Maternal Subjectivity Problem

Despite the theoretical developments of maternal studies and contemporary feminist psychoanalysis, the topics of maternal subjectivity and the embodied experience of being a mother continue to be marginalized in general psychoanalytic literature, debates, and training. Even as modern psychoanalysis transformed from a subject-object matrix to a subject-subject understanding (often referred to as "The Relational Turn"), talking about and listening to mothers is rarely done with privilege given namely to the maternal perspective, with the mother's subjectivity as the vantage point of narration. This approach is called a "matrifocal perspective" (O'Reilly, 2021) and stands in opposition to a daughter-centric approach where a mother's subjective experience is understood primarily from the context of her developmental history of being a daughter. It is somehow easier to see the daughter in the mother, thereby again returning to the perspective of the child, or focusing on how the mother is impacting her baby (Parker, 1995).

Baraitser (2012) has aptly pointed out that "motherhood brings feminist theory closest to its own blind spots" (p. 118). This is now acknowledged in feminist scholarship; the field has seen a development of theorizing maternal experience and agency (Bueskens, 2014), so much that its own branch is established as matricentric feminism (O'Reilly, 2007, 2021) which will be explored further in Chapter 3. In Baraitser's statement, feminist theory can be substituted with psychoanalysis. The question of the maternal holds a potential for bringing psychoanalysis further into intersubjective thinking. Indeed, the question of maternal subjectivity is the primary corroboration of Mitchell's (1974) claim that psychoanalysis and feminism are two forms of thinking that need each other. It is in feminist psychoanalysis we find the theoretical evolution towards seeing the mother as a subject in her own right and the acknowledgment of the child's need for the mother as a distinct subject in the development of intersubjective capacity (Benjamin, 1990; Hollway, 2001).

What is the problem then with the maternal subject? This is akin to asking what the problem is with the unconscious. By speaking to it, much is already lost. Winnicott's formulation of the baby that cannot exist without the mother, one of the earliest ideas of intersubjective thinking, directs us back to the mother, who also cannot exist without the baby. And yet she is the backdrop, the container, the proto-typical other, part- or whole-object, body parts, archetype, and "perhaps more than any subject position, [...] downright slippery" (Baraitser et al., 2009, para. 6). In psychoanalytic theory, she is most often conceptualized from the particular functions she fulfills for the child: "Motherhood connotes a natural state or condition which functions as an empty category into which children's needs can be placed." (Hollway, 2001, p. 1). "The maternal" has also been proposed to be the "foundation of the human condition" (Mayo & Moutsou, 2016, p. 3) in that it is the primary influence of how we live and situate ourselves culturally and relationally. Bueskens (2014) has argued that if we recognize the mother or "the maternal" as a valuable subject from which to generate knowledge, it may not only free women from the constraint of the institution of motherhood, but also shift our "epistemological, political, social, and psychic horizons" (p. 4).

The maternal subject is the event horizon of our inner object world. The mother is an "impossible" subject because of the universal bias we have when trying to appreciate her perspective, regardless of our own maternal status. She is both object to our needs and a subject in her own right, and the tension that this contradiction elicits is both a core existential conundrum of the human condition and crucial to the development of relational capacities (Benjamin, 1995). The maternal subject disrupts our very notion of subjectivity (Baraitser, 2009). Benjamin's (1995) theory of intersubjectivity demonstrates how the problem of maternal subjectivity constitutes an existential liability as "denial of the mother's subjectivity, in theory and in practice, profoundly impedes our ability to see the world as inhabited by equal subjects." (p. 31). From the intersubjective framework, exploration of maternal subjectivity addresses not only the lived experience of mothers, but also reaches into the area of understanding the fundamental nature of how we develop as relational beings.

The view of the woman as a separate subject is muddled when she becomes a mother, by herself and others. During pregnancy, she is not quite one nor two, and Stone (2014) has described how this puzzlement continues beyond delivery in that she is no longer automatically "recognized as a unified agent by others and can no longer easily regard herself as a unified agent either" (p. 325). The postpartum body changes interfere with our notion of subjectivity. McCarty (2020) has described the post-birth body as "an 'in-between' body, a liminal body subject to more nuanced readings of body image and corporeal ambiguity" (p. 38). Furman (1994) described how the maternal transition is characterized by ongoing shifts in body boundaries where the mother's process goes from investment of her child as a bodily part of herself to a gradual release of this and a transferring of bodily ownership back to the child. Mothering entails intense primitive states of fluid body-ego boundaries (Balsam, 2012; Furman, 1994). The anxiety symptoms related to this are easily pathologized which is problematic because they are developmental and evolutionary necessities. Mothers *rely* on flexibility in their body-ego boundaries in their normal narcissistic investment of their child that fuels attachment formation (Furman, 1994). This flexibility of body-ego boundaries relates to the profoundly coregulatory mode of interaction that characterizes the postpartum period which will be explored in Chapter 2 and Part II. In many aspects of life, narcissistic investment can take on purely mental forms, but relational investment in others, especially one's child, and especially if one has given birth to that child, has an acute somatic component.

It is this pressure on body boundaries that activates a woman's relational history in her maternal transition, for better and for worse, requiring the activation of defenses. The corporeal nature of mothering requires a unique flexibility and a reconfiguration of body boundaries, unlike any other time in life, challenging the idea of the subject as a physically and emotionally delineated entity. Pines (1978, 1994) focused on women's struggle towards individuality in light of the boundary pressures; she contended that pregnancy and motherhood can function psychologically as a work towards assertion of female subjectivity namely because of the maternal body transition because it is the ultimate concretization of separation from one's own mother. This notion points to the significant role of the physical experience of motherhood in the assertion of female subjectivity. Both Furman and Pines reached into the larger feminist critique of the Western patriarchal culture that offered the analysis of the maternal subjectivity problem as stemming from the way the individual is defined in contrast to the maternal. French feminists Kristeva (1987), Cixous (1976), and Irigaray (1987) analyzed the maternal as a powerful, yet highly conflictual subject position and the role of symbolic matricide as fundamental to patriarchal culture: The very notion of selfhood in Western culture is based on differentiation from the maternal body.

But how will more theorizing about the abstract question of the maternal make any difference in our clinical work with mothers? It likely will not, unless it has direct implications for our felt encounters with mothers and the way we relate to them in the therapy room. In modern relational psychoanalysis, we listen with our full subjectivity (Benjamin, 1990) and our bodies (Orbach, 2009). There has been a resurgence of general psychoanalytic interest in the body (e.g., Harrang et al., 2022), but it is contemporary feminist psychoanalysis focusing on maternal subjectivity that challenges us to consider how the clinical issues of working with mothers bring up the body in particular ways. Keeping in mind that embodiment is constitutive of subjectivity (Harrang et al., 2022) and that intersubjective relating builds on the foundation of somatic attunement as a prerequisite for mentalization processes (Hill, 2015), we must ask ourselves if we are equipped to listen to the deep layers of the experience of being and becoming a maternal body and subject, especially if the experience involves trauma? Because without the acknowledgment of the inherent problems with maternal embodied subjectivity, we risk reproducing the dynamics of othering and denying mothers' subjectivities which hinder healing. This is particularly problematic considering the disparities in Maternal Mental Health where women with any background or identity that deviates from institutionalized normative motherhood are disproportionately affected by PMADs and perinatal trauma (more on this in Chapter 3). Orbach (2006) warns us that "psychoanalysis' mentalist stance can fail to sufficiently address the subjective experience of the body as a body and in doing so can miss crucial dimensions of the patient's experience" (p. 89). We must begin with an acknowledgment of our inherent blind spots; the universal struggle of recognizing the mother as a full and *embodied* individual, as well as our inevitable unconscious projections onto her – and her body – when we sit across from her.

The feminist psychoanalytic approach is built on the assumptions that 1. the female body and female psychological development are inseparable and body changes in a woman's life are therefore integral to understanding her emotional life and thus maternal development (Balsam, 2012; Furman, 1982, 1994; Orbach, 2006, 2009; Pines, 1994), and 2. the maternal body is a site of inevitable conflict, concretely and symbolically (Stone, 2014), and therefore highly exposed to othering and the impact of trauma. In previous writings, I have explored these assumptions by analyzing the body fantasies and their functions and emphasizing the maternal body as the main site for the processing of intrapsychic and interpersonal meanings (Vissing, 2015). My analysis led me to conclude that it is not sufficient to only address the question of maternal subjectivity. The "problem" of the maternal body is key to the question of understanding maternal subjectivity and how the feminist psychoanalytic approach can inform and transform our clinical work with mothers. In short, the "problem" with the maternal subject is her body. The way her embodiment disrupts our usual understanding of the delineated subject makes her identity "non-conforming". But the body is also the solution to finding our way back to her, as a full subject in her own right, untied from institutionalized patriarchal motherhood.

The Maternal Body Problem and Trauma

Stone (2014) contends that the problem of selfhood being defined in opposition to the maternal is directly related to the maternal body: "Ultimately, what we are expected to separate from is the whole field of maternal body relations: The realm of intimate mother-infant dependency in which flows and exchanges of affect and bodily energy take place" (p. 327). The sense of self for the new mother is a particularly challenging achievement because of the paradox of embodying a new maternal self while embodying a relational realm that is perceived as the contrast to selfhood. The newness of the maternal body can be a rich, fulfilling, and pleasurable experience, but the loss of sense of self that is widely recognized as part of the maternal transition is also a bodily loss with everything that entails grief. In her analysis of maternal desire, de Marneffe (2004) has pointed out that when we internalize the discourses of motherhood being antithetical to self, it profoundly impacts our ability to recognize and experience maternal desires as positive aspects of self. It is the characteristics of the female body that make it elusive and incoherent from the perspective of patriarchy, which makes it "an undecidable space that lacks a coherent identity and is always subject to flux" (Mayo & Moutsou, 2016, p. 5). McCarthy (2020) has described the postpartum state as "unknown fleshy subjectivity" (p. 42). The significant material changes in the body during pregnancy and postpartum can elicit any thinkable emotional reaction, including positive experiences and sensations. But regardless of how positive these changes are experienced they mark a radical transformation of the body-self that heightens existential vulnerability. The corporeal condition of giving birth involves a paradox: It establishes a new subjectivity while also disturbing the sense of being a subject: "The body becomes a kind of subjective object, mine but not mine, functioning, but not as I know it, an unfamiliar vehicle in which to navigate a new material landscape" (McCarthy, 2020, p. 44). The destabilization of the body-self in the postpartum can push a mother into dissociation where the mind and body feel disconnected. Body and self can seem divorced from each other – which is exactly what happens in trauma.

Trauma deeply impacts the sense of self. While it might be an interesting philosophical discussion, it would be of questionable clinical value to discuss whether this destabilization of selfhood and the bodily reorganization of self that the maternal transition causes constitute a form of trauma in itself. It is instead my primary concern to consider the experiences of women who go through the perinatal transition with a trauma history. The maternal transition and trauma both cause significant destabilization, in intertwined psychological and somatic ways, where the body-self undergoes dramatic upheaval. This intertwining of trauma and the seismic identity shift of motherhood is further complicated by the fact that symptoms of trauma (and other mental health conditions like depression and anxiety) and symptoms of pregnancy and postpartum overlap and are not discernible. Fatigue, sleep disturbances, hyperarousal, digestion issues, breathing issues, and general dysregulation without a clear cause can all manifest from trauma or the physiological adaptations of pregnancy, or both. From a social perspective, destabilization of the sense of self is also exacerbated by the experience of being othered (Agarwal, 2021), adding a layer of strain to mothers who are othered because of aspects of their identity, for example, ethnicity and racial identity, sexual orientation, immigration status, socioeconomic status, disability status, marital status, etc., which will be elaborated in Chapter 3.

Mothering from a Traumatized Body Self

The experience of being a body-self is formed in the relational matrix of embodiment (LaPierre, 2015; Orbach, 2006, 2009), which anchors our identity formation to a bodily foundation (Caldwell, 2016). Our perception of our bodies are outcomes of the intimate relationship we make with our surroundings (Orbach, 2011). Of the many ways we are impacted by trauma, the impact on our somatically anchored and relationally developed self is arguably the most profound. Here trauma impinges on exactly that which is crucial to mothering and the maternal transition: An integrated embodied sense of self. Relational trauma can cause a sense of bodylessness (Caldwell, 2018) or "body insecurity" as described by Orbach (2006): "Where the body has been welcomed, treated in a consistent manner, its gestures mirrored, and so on, the sense that the body is stable and sure will prevail. Where the relation to the body has been unstable and inconsistent, or when the body's gesture has gone unrecognized, then this instability will operate like a fixed structure" (p. 92). Paraphrasing Winnicott's idea of the false self, Orbach (2006) also introduces the idea of the false body, which is a sense of body-self created in the absence of a relation to a "true" body. Just as the false self develops from adapting to the caregiver's responses at the expense of the development of the true self, the bodily self forms into a "false body" characterized by body insecurity. At the core of the false body-self is the experience of only feeling alive when recovering from states of crisis. Body insecurity is thus not only a state of an insecure body self but also a lack of bodily felt sense of self. The body is not only impacted by trauma but becomes the "place of remembered trauma" (Orbach, 2006, p. 95). This somatic sting of trauma on the bodily sense of self is particularly grave in the perinatal context where the maternal body is the site of transformation and the struggle for assertion of a unique new form of subjectivity.

Caldwell (2018) identifies the four characteristics of bodylessness to be: Ignoring the body, seeing the body as an object or project, hating the body, and making one's own or other's bodies wrong. Considering body insecurity in the perinatal context, the problem of maternal embodied subjectivity can be seen as a problem of bodylessness, exacerbated by the ways the maternal body is objectified and evaluated by the biomedical stance of obstetrics and patriarchal motherhood (this will be elaborated in Chapter 3). Ignoring the body, which often happens through numbing or dissociation as an autonomic somatic survival response to overwhelm, puts the new mother in a dire situation as she relies on her sensations and felt experience to regulate her baby and herself. When the stress and anxiety of the body changes of the perinatal period interact with trauma reactions, varying degrees of bodylessness follow. Bodyless mothering or mothering from the "false" body is a relational trauma state; not only does it entail a state of body insecurity and destabilization of the self, but it also hinders the discovery and assertion of the new body self of the mother's embodied relational subjectivity. The psychosocial dynamics of maternal bodylessness will be discussed further in Chapter 3.

When we conceptualize the maternal transition from psychoanalytic, trauma-focused, and somatic psychology approaches, we acknowledge the exacerbation of the destabilization of the body-self that trauma causes and its devastating impact on the mother. The vulnerability of the sense of self in the postpartum is intensified by the destabilization of self that trauma causes – and vice versa. This two-fold vulnerability is integral to the "problem" of maternal subjectivity, and the corporeal nature of both the maternal transition and trauma make it a body-related matter. The mother who carries a trauma history or who experiences trauma in her maternal transition (or both) is therefore twice exposed, double-whammied. Her trauma reactions are exacerbated by the physicality of the maternal transition and its somatic vulnerability, and her experience of her maternal transition is colored by her trauma history. She needs care and treatment that addresses the magnitude of this convergence of somatic pressures.

It All Comes Back to the (Maternal) Body: How Relational Psychoanalysis Brings the Body into Perinatal Clinical Work

As shown, contemporary feminist psychoanalytic thinking points us to the importance of the body for therapy during the perinatal period. Maternal subjectivity is a subject position that is uniquely embodied and relational as well as deeply conflictual, with or without a trauma history. This explains why mothers are particularly exposed to the impacts of trauma as they go through the maternal transition, and even more so if they are exposed to systemic dynamics of othering. It also means we cannot appreciate mothers fully in the therapeutic relationship without dedicated clinical attention to the embodied and relational aspects of the experience of mothering, including how this impacts the therapeutic relationship. The complex connections between conscious and unconscious material of the maternal transition are played out in and through the maternal body, both experientially through sensations and through body-related meaning-making.

When we appreciate psychodynamic thinking of maternal embodied relational subjectivity, several intertwined points inform our interventions. Firstly, the inherent issues with maternal subjectivity make a heavy emphasis on the assertion of subjectivity a necessity. A sense of maternal self cannot be taken for granted; it is achieved through the psychological struggles related to the experience of having become a maternal body and how that is conflictual considering Western culture's view of selfhood as oppositional to the maternal position. Interventions must be formed so they facilitate this process of asserting maternal subjectivity on nonverbal and verbal levels. Secondly, the body boundary problem makes it necessary to work with both body meanings and experientially with experiences of being and having a maternal body, in this struggle towards claiming maternal embodied subjectivity. These two are deeply intertwined in that maternal subjectivity cannot be meaningfully addressed outside of its embodied experience; having and being a maternal body is the foundation of maternal subjectivity (Stone, 2014). These points are furthered by the impacts of trauma; the loosening of the body ego and body boundaries of the maternal transition makes the period highly vulnerable to the destabilization of embodied subjectivity that trauma causes.

Feminist psychoanalytic thinking shows us that sensitive therapeutic work in the perinatal period must be somatically relational to capture how the corporeal reality of the maternal transition is fundamental to its ontology. We must speak to and with maternal subjectivity by finding our way to the maternal body. We must listen to maternal development as it manifests in the body (Balsam, 2012). The implications of a full appreciation of maternal embodied subjectivity must involve clinical sensitivity to the physical aspects of maternal subjectivity and therefore somatic communications in the therapeutic process. This is corroborated by the intersubjective insight from affect regulation research that "we sense our subjectivity and the subjectivity of others through the ebbs and flows of arousal that course through our bodies and theirs" (Hill, 2015, p. 9). Including the bodily countertransferential experiences helps therapists develop a fuller understanding of the client's bodily development (Orbach, 2006). A somatic intersubjective approach must therefore support the mother in discovering, integrating, and claiming her new maternal subjectivity in an embodied relational way, beyond the limitations of verbal work, as opposed to a purely verbal and cognitive process.

A consequence of this for the therapeutic relationship is that we must acknowledge the challenges of the particular somatic transferential field when working in the perinatal period, especially with trauma. This requires us to develop a tolerance for sitting with the intense forms of dysregulation that the maternal transition and trauma engenders, to work in the therapeutic resonance of attending to the somatic transference and countertransference (Orbach, 2006, 2009), and to help our perinatal clients build the capacity for somatic receptivity while appreciating how that it is particularly difficult given the vulnerability of the perinatal transition. The normal fluidity of body-ego states and body boundaries that mothering requires (Furman, 1994) makes it easy to pathologize the dysregulation of the perinatal period. Here it is a significant advantage of the feminist psychoanalytic approach that it prevents pathologizing of the dysregulation of the perinatal transition because of the developmental and philosophical understanding of the inherent struggles of embodied relational maternal subjectivity. Orbach's model of affording value to bodily felt experiences of the transferential work and "scrutinizing [...] the corporeal intersubjectivity" (2006, p. 97) is highly relevant for working with the new mother. It is a way to acknowledge the body's subjectivity and intersubjectivity.

Our bodies receive the "body-to-body relational mismatching" of our clients' intersubjective history (Orbach, 2006, p. 100). From this intersubjective understanding, Orbach (2006) contends that our work must be oriented towards helping our clients experience that they have bodies; to discover the interrelatedness of their subjectivity and embodiment. Working experientially and relationally towards cultivating an embodied sense of self is not only crucial for trauma treatment with mothers, but also carries an added layer of challenge due to the ontological and intersubjective issues of maternal embodied subjectivity discussed in this chapter. The maternal transition can be seen as a struggle to rediscover one's embodiment. How do we help our clients transition into having and being maternal bodies? This requires the therapist to first accept and tolerate the dysregulation coming from the two-fold upheaval of the sense of self that the maternal transition and trauma cause. Working with the client towards discovering, verbalizing, and expressing the new maternal body self cannot be rushed or forced without adequate relational work of attunement to this dysregulation. This is not merely attuning to emotional distress or sympathetic arousal understood as stressors to adapt to; it is to attune to the existential destabilization of the sense of being an embodied and clearly defined subject. The common phrase "when a baby is born so is a mother" not only points to the understanding of the new maternal role being added to the mother's identity; understood somatically, the maternal transition brings a woman back to the ontological realm of arriving into her subjectivity through the body that we all begin life from (what Orbach (2006) calls the preintegrated body). We must first work to establish body coherence (Orbach, 2006) before we can build body narrative and from there a bodyfully anchored sense of self; our body identity (Caldwell, 2016). This clinical strategy must be applied with acute sensitivity to how the nature of mothering makes it a challenging and fragmented process to achieve coherence in one's new maternal body narrative, even more so in the context of body insecurity and bodylessness caused by trauma.

On the question of whether a psychoanalytic approach is compatible with somatic psychology, it is important to note that bodily focused psychotherapy has been influenced by relational psychoanalysis and vice versa, in mutually enriching ways (LaPierre, 2015). Rolef Ben-Shahar (2014) notes that it was the relational turn in psychoanalysis that facilitated the flourishing of body psychotherapy in the general field of psychotherapy due to the shift away from the classic stance of neutrality and therapeutic objectivity. The relational developments of psychoanalysis have evolved from the integration of research findings from interpersonal neurobiology and affect theory (Hill, 2015) that bodily focused psychotherapy is based on. Furthermore, the psychoanalytic understandings of the intertwining of female embodiment and female psychological development (Balsam, 2012) and how this makes the maternal transition above all a bodily identity development (Furman, 1994), are paralleled by the body psychotherapy understanding of identity as "generated and lived out in the body" and the assumptions that working consciously with bodily identity is crucial for healing and empowerment. (Caldwell, 2016, p. 221). The contemporary developments in psychoanalysis have also brought the body into focus with an interest in what the body is needing in its own right, instead of the previous analytic approach of only addressing the symbolic meanings of somatic symptoms (Orbach, 2009). The integration of psychodynamic psychotherapy and somatic psychology will also be addressed in Chapter 4.

Maternal identity development has largely been seen as a primarily mental and cognitive construct in mainstream clinical psychology, but with the feminist developments of psychoanalytic thinking and the advances of somatic psychology, we can now acknowledge its somatic intersubjective foundations and form our clinical work with mothers accordingly. When assertion of maternal embodied subjectivity is done within the therapeutic containment of the intersubjective psychoanalytic approach combined with somatic resonance and attunement (Chapter 5), the complex interplay between the nonverbal and verbal levels of experience of the maternal transition can be acknowledged clinically by simultaneously building sensory awareness and facilitating the discovery and vocabulary of maternal body identity and narrative (Chapter 6). Thus, the foundation is laid for safe trauma resolution in the perinatal context (Chapter 7) and creative and holistic treatment planning (Chapter 8).

References

Agarwal, P. (2021). *(M)otherhood. On the choices of being a woman.* Canongate Books.

Balsam, R.H. (2012). *Women's bodies in psychoanalysis.* Routledge. 10.4324/9780203078327

Baraitser, L. (2009). *Maternal encounters: The ethics of interruptions.* Routledge.

Baraitser, L. (2012). Communality across time: Responding to encounters with maternal encounters: The ethics of interruptions. *Studies in Gender and Sexuality, 13*(2), 117–122. 10.1080/15240657.2012.682932

Baraitser, L., Spigel, S., Betterton, R., Curk, R., Hollway, W., Jensen, T., & Tyler, I. (2009). Mapping maternal subjectivities, identities, and ethics. *Studies in the Maternal, 1*(1). Retrieved from https://www.mamsie.bbk.ac.uk/articles/10.16995/sim.170/

Benjamin, J. (1990). An outline of intersubjectivity: The development of recognition. *Psychoanalytic Psychology, 7*, 33–46. 10.1037/h0085258

Benjamin, J. (1995). *Like subjects, love objects: Essays on recognition and sexual difference.* University Press.

Bibring, G.L. (1959). Some considerations of the psychological processes in pregnancy. *Psychoanalytic Study of the Child, 14*, 113–121. 10.1080/00797308.1959.11822824

Bibring, G.L., Dwyer, T.F., Huntington, D.S., & Valenstein, A.F. (1961). A study of the psychological processes in pregnancy and of the earliest mother-child relationship. *Psychoanalytic Study of the Child, 16*, 9–72. 10.1080/00797308.1961.11823197

Blum, L. (2007). Psychodynamics of postpartum depression. *Psychoanalytic Psychology, 24*(1), 45–62. 10.1037/0736-9735.24.1.45

Bueskens, P. (2014). *Mothering and psychoanalysis. Clinical, sociological, and feminist perspectives*. Demeter Press.

Caldwell, C.M. (2016). Body identity development: Definitions and discussions. *Body, Movement and Dance in Psychotherapy, 11*(4), 220–234. 10.1080/17432979.2016.1145141

Caldwell, C.M. (2018). *Bodyfulness. Somatic practices for presence, empowerment, and waking up in this life*. Shambala.

Cixous, H. (1976). The laugh of the medusa. *Signs, 1*(4), 875–893. 10.1086/493306

de Marneffe, D. (2004). *Maternal desire: On children, love, and the inner life*. Time Warner Book Group.

Deutsch, H. (1945). *The psychology of women*, Vol. II. Bantam Books.

Freud, S. (1932). Female sexuality. *International Journal of Psycho-Analysis, 13*, 281–298.

Freud, S. (1933). New introductory lectures on psychoanalysis. Lecture 33: Femininity. In J. Strachey (Ed.) (1961), *The standard edition of the complete psychological works of Sigmund Freud* (pp. 136–157). The Hogarth Press.

Furman, E. (1982). Mothers have to be there to be left. *The Psychoanalytic Study of the Child, 37*, 15–28. 10.1080/00797308.1982.11823356

Furman, E. (1994). Early aspects of mothering: What makes it so hard to be there to be left. *Journal of Child Psychotherapy, 20*(2), 149–164. 10.1080/00754179408256746

Harrang, C., Tillotson, D., & Winters, N.C. (2022). General introduction. In C. Harrang, D. Tillotson, & N.C. Winters (Eds.), *Body as psychoanalytic object. Clinical applications from Winnicott to Bion and beyond* (pp. 1–9). Routledge. 10.4324/9781003195559

Hill, D. (2015). *Affect regulation theory. A clinical model*. Norton.

Hollway, W. (2001). From motherhood to maternal subjectivity. *International Journal of Critical Psychology, 2*, 13–38.

Irigaray, L. (1987). *Sexes and Genealogies*. Columbia University Press.

Kleiman, K. (2017). *The art of holding in therapy: An essential intervention for postpartum depression and anxiety*. Routledge.

Kristeva, J. (1987). *Tales of love: European perspectives*. Columbia University Press.

LaPierre, A. (2015). Relational body psychotherapy (or relational somatic psychology). *International Body Psychotherapy Journal, 14*(2), 80–100.

Mahler, M.S., Pine, F., & Bergman, A. (1975). *The psychological birth of the human infant*. Basic Books.

Mayo, R., & Moutsou, C. (Eds.). (2016). *The mother in psychoanalysis and beyond*. Routledge. 10.4324/9781315715308

McCarthy, J. (2020). The corporeal dimensions of motherhood. In C. Arnold-Baker (Ed.), *The existential crisis of motherhood* (pp. 37–55). Palgrave Macmillan.

Menken, A. (2008). A psychodynamic approach to treatment for postpartum depression. In S.S. Dowd, & A.E. Menken (Eds.), *Perinatal and postpartum mood disorders: Perspectives and treatment guide for the health care practitioner* (pp. 309–320). Springer.

Mitchell, J. (1974). *Psychoanalysis and feminism*. Pantheon Books.

O'Reilly, A. (2007). Feminist mothering. In A. O'Reilly (Ed.), *Maternal theory. Essential readings* (p. 792–821). Demeter Press.

O'Reilly, A. (2021). *Matricentric feminism. Theory, activism, practice. The 2nd edition*. Demeter Press. 10.2307/j.ctv1k2j331

Orbach, S. (2006). How can we have a body?: Desires and corporeality. *Studies In Gender & Sexuality, 7*(1), 89–111.

Orbach, S. (2009). *Bodies*. Picador.

Orbach, S. (2011). Losing Bodies. *Social Research, 78*(2), 387–394.

Parker, R. (1995). *Mother love/mother hate*. BasicBooks.

Pines, D. (1978). On becoming a parent. *International Journal of Child Psychology, 4*(4), 19–31.

Pines, D. (1982). The relevance of early psychic development to pregnancy and abortion. *International Journal of Psychoanalysis, 63*, 311–319.

Pines, D. (1994). *A woman's unconscious use of her body*. Yale University Press.

Rolef Ben-Shahar, A. (2014). *Touching the relational edge*. Routledge. 10.4324/9780429484100

Stone, A. (2014). Psychoanalysis and maternal subjectivity. In P. Bueskens (Ed.), *Mothering and psychoanalysis: Clinical, sociological, and feminist perspectives* (pp. 325–342). Demeter Press.

Vissing, H. (2015). The triumph over the body: Body fantasies and their protective function. *Journal of the Motherhood Initiative for Research and Community Involvement*, 6(1), 168–175.

2

Understanding Trauma in Light of the Biological Changes of Motherhood

"Mommy Brain" Revisited: Trauma-Informed Understanding of the Biological Adaptations of the Maternal Transition

We are only beginning to understand the neurobiological complexities of the perinatal transition and know little about how trauma impacts this vulnerable period. An emerging body of literature has demonstrated that endocrine systems (in particular oxytocin and cortisol), neurological systems (e.g., hippocampal structures and the Hypothalamic-Pituitary-Adrenal (HPA) axis), and immune systems (catecholamine and inflammatory responses) undergo dramatic and intertwined reorganizing in pregnancy, lactation, and postpartum (Kendall-Tackett, 2017a). Although general neuroscience has shown that the socioemotional brain remains plastic throughout the lifespan (Hill, 2015), the neurological adaptations of the perinatal transition are so significant that the term "maternal brain plasticity" has been established (Kim & Strathearn, 2016). Reproduction-related plasticity involves brain regions related to reward and motivation, threat detection, self-regulation, social cognition, and empathy (Barba-Müller et al., 2019) and possibly reflects a pruning of the maternal brain for caregiving specialization (Iyengar et al., 2019). Beck et al. (2013) have even called pregnancy "a biochemical storm or assault" (p. 82).

These changes, and the plasticity of the maternal brain, are *experience-dependent*: Endocrine factors activate neural circuits that are then maintained by experiential factors in the interactions with the baby. The neurobiological adaptations of the maternal brain continue to change through the postpartum period. This is most evident in lactation, but is also seen in the attachment-building process, likely as a reflection of the ongoing adaptations to the development of the child, or a "build-up" of the capacities over time (Barba-Müller et al., 2019). Similarly, the maternal brain adaptations must be understood in the context of the mother's neurological developmental history – essentially a mother's trauma and resiliency history. Indeed, the challenges of the maternal transition become heightened with early-life adversities, unresolved trauma, or psychopathology (Iyengar et al., 2019).

How Trauma is Nuancing Our Understanding of Oxytocin

Several behavioral phenomena related to motherhood have been illuminated by neuroendocrinology research. In particular, the importance of oxytocin for the mother-child bond is well-documented and oxytocin plays an important role far beyond uterine contractions and milk ejection (Kim & Strathearn, 2016; Uvnäs-Moberg, 2014). Insights about these neurobiological aspects of the maternal transition continue to inspire development of more effective clinical interventions (Kim & Strathearn, 2016), for example how we can create more "oxytocic" environments for new mothers through relational and trauma-informed support (Kendall-Tackett, 2019). However, the role of trauma has nuanced our understanding of this: Using oxytocin pharmacologically has not been shown to be universally effective and sometimes causes paradoxical effects, particularly for people with disrupted attachment history (Kim & Strathearn, 2016).

Increased oxytocin following birth enables mothers to be highly attuned to social cues, so they provide optimal care for their babies (Uvnäs-Moberg, 2014). But this situation also creates a challenge of increased sensitivity to misattunements from the surroundings (Kendall-Tackett, 2019). The understanding of oxytocin as universally positive for social functioning is therefore undergoing revisions towards a more nuanced and arguably more trauma-informed view that its "primary mechanism of action may lie in increasing the salience of social cues" (Kim & Strathearn, 2016, p. 67). Research on the oxytocin system have in this way shown that the "perinatal period is a unique opportunity to recognize trauma and its effects" (Kendall-Tackett, 2017b, p. 150). Neuroendocrine adaptations of motherhood, such as oxytocin-mediated processes, are highly complex and interact with a woman's attachment history. Research demonstrates that variations in the oxytocin systems predict individual differences in adaptations to motherhood (Kim & Strathearn, 2016). The individual's history of early-life adversity or trauma and insecure attachment are considered important factors that impact the oxytocin-related adaptations of the maternal transition. The oxytocic state helps mothers, but also makes them vulnerable. It is crucial for clinicians to be mindful of the delicate biological aspects of these adaptations. Understanding oxytocin research helps clinicians be diligent in our relational work to avoid and prevent misattunements with the new mother client with a trauma history.

The Overlap Between Perinatal Changes, PMADs, and Trauma Biology: HPA Axis Dysregulation and Inflammation

PMADs have unique neural profiles during the postpartum period compared with depression and anxiety disorders occurring at other times in a woman's life (Pawluski et al., 2017). Neuroscientific studies of the maternal brain have shown that the previously discussed "maternal plasticity" – the vast neural plasticity specific to reproduction – likely confers a vulnerability for mental health issues in certain contexts (Barba-Müller et al., 2019).

Integrating findings from psychoneuroimmunology, the study of biological stress responses, has been crucial in shedding light on the complex links between stress, inflammatory responses, and postpartum depression (Kendall-Tackett, 2017a) – and trauma. Both general depression research (Lee & Giuliani, 2019), research on PMADs (Kendall-Tackett, 2017a), and research on trauma (Quinones et al., 2020) have identified increased inflammatory activation as a key etiological factor. The perinatal period carries an inherent risk in the natural elevation of proinflammatory cytokines in the third trimester (Kendall-Tackett, 2017a). Pregnant and postpartum women, therefore, have a heightened vulnerability to the inflammation-depression dynamic because pregnancy naturally causes inflammation levels to rise. Inflammation has been linked to depression in several ways, including its impact on the HPA axis causing dysregulation of cortisol and its impact on serotonin. Another significant factor here is sleep, as sleep disturbances are experienced by the body as inflammatory-inducing stress. Sleep and depression are bidirectionally related: "Sleep disturbance increases depression risk and depression causes sleep problems" (Kendall-Tackett, 2010, p. 8). The delicate interactions between inflammatory responses and the HPA axis are a factor in postpartum mood (Duthie & Reynolds, 2013). However, we cannot understand these interactions without considering the role of trauma, as PMADs have high comorbidity with trauma. 65% of perinatal women with PTSD also present with PPD (Grisbrook & Letourneau, 2021).

The primary physiological reaction to stress and trauma is the activation of the sympathetic nervous system, HPA axis, and inflammatory response system (Kingston & Mughal, 2020). Stress and depression are linked in complex ways, yet still distinct. Dysregulation of the HPA axis is linked to depression, possibly in a causal way. Both pregnancy and trauma strain the HPA axis functioning significantly, making the expecting or new mother with a trauma history highly vulnerable to mood disturbances from a biological perspective. Stress also activates the inflammatory response system, which increases the risk of mood disorders (Bergink et al., 2014). Trauma increases this risk further. The amount of evidence linking maternal stress, trauma, and PMADs has researchers recommending standard stress screening (Kingston & Mughal, 2020; Venta et al., 2021) and trauma screening (Grisbrook & Letourneau, 2021; Padin et al., 2022).

Traumatic Childbirth

From a trauma-informed approach, it is hard to overestimate the significance of childbirth. As the review of the wide range of perinatal trauma in Introduction to Part I demonstrated, we cannot solely focus on traumatic childbirth in trauma-informed Maternal Mental Health. However, we must recognize that traumatic childbirth is a central and cyclonic point of impact from which we can expand and nuance our clinical thinking. Research on traumatic childbirth has explored its complex dynamics, risk factors, and consequences. Beck (2015) developed a middle-range theory that demonstrates "the ever-widening ripple effect" of traumatic childbirth: Mothers suffer long-term chronic consequences of a traumatic birth including its impact on breastfeeding and subsequent childbirths. The clinical language related to traumatic childbirth is a good example of paradigmatic thinking that limits our knowledge about trauma in the perinatal period. The term trauma in medical settings usually means physiological injury, which in obstetric contexts refers to emergency cesarean, postpartum hemorrhaging, perineal lacerations, or injury to internal organs, etc. This language is part of effective obstetric care, but it carries a risk of overlooking the emotional and mental health aspects related to the medical events of childbirth. One important insight of trauma-informed care is that psychological trauma is subjective (Beck, 2015). That trauma is a subjective experience has been widely acknowledged in the general trauma literature for decades (Levine, 2010). Beck's (2015) research has demonstrated a common theme of experiencing being dismissed in narratives of women who experienced traumatic childbirth.

Although traumatic childbirth is an issue of global concern, there are differences in prevalence across different countries. Some studies comparing countries have demonstrated a correlation between lower rates of birth interventions and lower rates of birth trauma for both mothers and providers (Kendall-Tackett, 2017a; Kendall-Tackett & Beck, 2022). Increasing medical interventions may increase the risks of birth trauma, especially in the case of the mother having a history of previous trauma. A key variable, however, is the mother's relationship with her provider during birth.

Women with PTSD in pregnancy were more like to have had exposures to childhood abuse and prior traumatic reproductive event, to have cumulative sociodemographic risk factors, comorbid depression, and anxiety, and to have sought mental health treatment in the past (Seng et al., 2009). Ayers et al. (2016) note that trauma history interacts with birth interventions to increase the risk of PTSD after birth. Conversely, support during birth can mitigate the relationship between previous trauma and birth-related PTSD; as well as the relationship between birth intervention and postpartum PTSD (Ford & Ayers, 2011). Research on the links between medical interventions and the mother's subjective experience may help us understand trauma in the context of the maternal transition. The cumulative effects of previous trauma and medical complications and interventions during childbirth can create significant rippling between the medical and psychological effects. Clinicians must address both.

Connecting the Dots: The Causal Loops of Perinatal Trauma and Reproductive Biology

We have yet to discover much about the biological aspects of trauma in the perinatal period and how they interact with psychological and social factors, but the available research informs plausible theories on causal loops and interactions. The delicate interactions between inflammatory responses and the HPA axis are established factors in PMADs as well as trauma. Stress and trauma cause inflammatory responses and endocrine dysregulation likely disrupting the normal inflammatory adjustments of the perinatal period, likely contributing to PMADs (Chen & Lacey, 2018; Finy & Christian, 2018).

It is less clear how maternal brain plasticity interacts and overlaps with trauma. However, it is established knowledge that an individual's own trauma history, particularly early adverse experiences, is linked to physiological sequelae like allostatic load, autoimmune illnesses, and other health issues that are inflammation-linked conditions, which again are linked to Mental Health disorders like depression and anxiety (Bergink et al., 2014; Danese et al., 2009; Kendall-Tackett, 2007). Systemic contexts of health inequity and discrimination exacerbate and are intertwined with individual allostatic load and trauma history (this will be addressed in Chapter 3). A mother's trauma history can interact with the impact of medical interventions to increase the risks of traumatic childbirth, which can affect postpartum adjustment. Inspired by Beck's (2015) use of the causal loop model for traumatic childbirth, Figure 2.1 shows possible causal loops of perinatal trauma and its interaction with the biology of reproduction and its relation to PMADs. This causal loop model is useful for shifting Maternal Mental Health towards trauma-informed clinical thinking that integrates our current knowledge from psychoneuroimmunology research. It is aimed to assist us in answering the question: What are the implications for the treatment of PMADs and trauma in the perinatal period considering the biomedical research? Aligned with the philosophy of complexity theory, this model acknowledges that it is often impossible to know all contributors, influences, and factors, and yet it is still an analysis valuable for informing clinical practice. Furthermore, it may buffer the unrealistic expectation that we can know and control all factors (Borrell-Carrió et al., 2004).

Implications for Trauma-Responsive Maternal Mental Health: Fighting Inflammation with Stress-Reduction and Adopting a Plasticity Perspective

The neuroscientific insights about the biology of PMADs, and the significant impact of trauma on the maternal brain and nervous

86 ♦ Overview of Trauma in the Perinatal Period

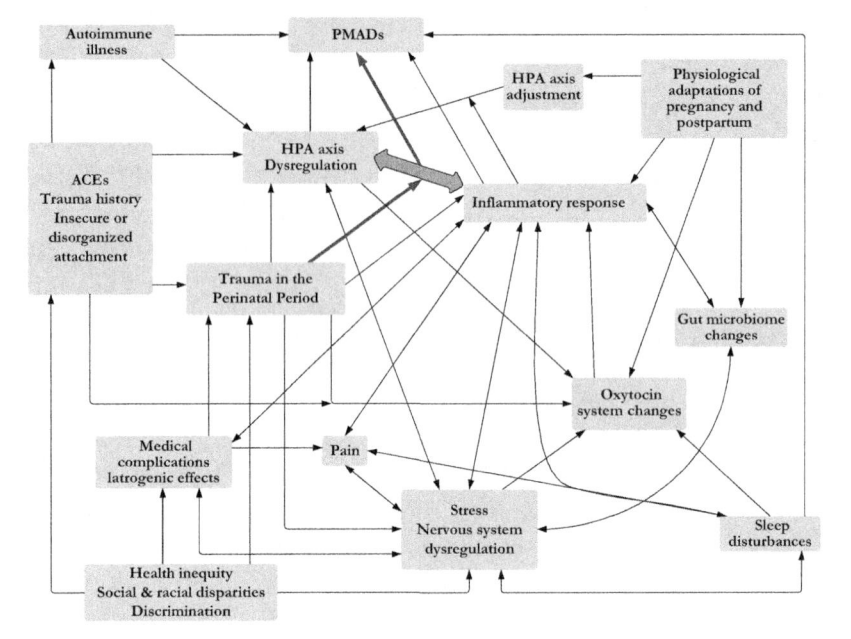

FIGURE 2.1 Causal Loops of Trauma and PMADs

system, inform clinical work in two ways: First, we must realize the magnitude of the sequelae of trauma due to the vulnerabilities of the perinatal transition, and second, we must seize the promising opportunities for healing given the plasticity that comes with the maternal transition. Neuroscience and psychoneuroimmunology research indicate that trauma-informed treatment must include an element of anti-inflammatory intervention (Gill et al., 2020). This includes stress reduction (Kendall-Tackett, 2010). As mentioned, pregnant and postpartum women are already at increased risk for depression, but when we add the impact of trauma to this, which also includes dysregulation of the HPA axis, the sensitive biology of the perinatal transition is strained even further. Oxytocin, released during labor, milk ejection, and skin-to-skin contact can counter many of these stress effects, but it also increases mothers' vulnerability because of their heightened sensitivity to social cues (Uvnäs-Moberg, 2014). Stress can also suppress oxytocin, increasing breastfeeding difficulties and compromising the mother's mental health (Kendall-Tackett et al., 2015; Uvnäs-Moberg, 2014).

In their review article, Kingston and Mughal (2020) found that infants who were held and touched more by their mothers who suffered from prenatal depression did not have the same adverse effects compared with infants who received less maternal care. They point out the potential for healing:

> On a clinical level, these studies provide a basis for encouragement for pregnant women struggling with anxiety or depression. The emerging evidence that stroking an infant can moderate the effect of prenatal depression on child outcomes is a hopeful message of a powerful, doable maternal intervention.
> (Kingston & Mughal, 2020, p. 21)

Research findings like these inform clinical intervention. From a somatic therapy perspective, touch resonates fully with the principles of improving nervous system regulation and facilitating trauma resolution through coregulation. However, as with all perinatal interventions, it must be used in a way that considers the mother's experience and perspective, rather than as a directive (this will be addressed in Chapters 5 and 6 on how to facilitate therapeutic safety and cultivate sensory awareness in perinatal psychotherapy).

Although psychotherapy and similar psychosocial support interventions do not involve nutrition or medication that targets inflammation, stress reduction offers a crucial anti-inflammatory component of holistic care. The inflammatory response is strongly associated with stress, sleep disturbances, and pain (Kendall-Tackett, 2017a). Inflammation is not only the driving biological mechanism of the negative outcomes of stress; it is also exacerbated by a lack of social support (Uchino et al., 2018). Conversely, social support and secure attachments are considered to have anti-inflammatory effects (Uchino et al., 2018; Venta et al., 2021). Nervous system regulation is a potent way to reduce the stress patterns of inflammation. Somatic work targets the underlying causes of inflammation by addressing the nervous system dysregulation-stress patterns. Dysregulating behavioral patterns related to trauma and toxic stress that reinforce stress and inflammatory responses can be targeted clinically in this way. Additionally, somatic techniques that support clients in their social functioning by working with them in a coregulating way can increase the regulating effects of social support. The somatic clinical techniques of resonance, coregulation, and sensory awareness will be presented in Chapters 5–7. Considerations for anti-inflammatory holistic treatment planning will be presented in Chapter 8.

The research on attachment trauma and its connection to perinatal biological changes is sobering, but also points to crucial hope for healing. Iyengar et al. (2019) concluded from their study that mothers with unresolved trauma do not need to fully reach the stage of earned security to mitigate the intergenerational impacts of trauma, but that the continued process of reorganizing towards secure attachment makes a significant difference. Thus, it is not necessary for a new mother to have completely resolved her own attachment trauma to circumvent the intergenerational transmission of misattunement patterns in her relationship with her child. If she is "attachment reorganizing," and if the care she receives is attuned and trauma-sensitive, the relationship with her child can become one of security and she can work towards asserting her new maternal subjectivity. Although brain research shows altered activity in the maternal brain systems in mothers with unresolved trauma, we must balance this with our knowledge of the potential for life-long neuroplasticity (Kingston & Mughal, 2020) and trauma healing (Levine, 2010). A trauma history is not deterministic. Although a significant effort is needed, the delicate biological aspects of trauma in the perinatal period can be treated.

References

Ayers, S., Bond, R., Bertullies, S., & Wijma, K. (2016). The aetiology of post-traumatic stress following childbirth: A meta-analysis and theoretical framework. *Psychological Medicine*, 46(6), 1121–1134. 10.1017/S0033291715002706

Barba-Müller, E., Craddock, S., Carmona, S., & Hoekzema, E. (2019). Brain plasticity in pregnancy and the postpartum period: Links to maternal caregiving and mental health. *Archives of Women's Mental Health, 22*, 289–299. 10.1007/s00737-018-0889-z

Beck, C.T. (2015). Middle range theory of traumatic childbirth: The ever-widening ripple effect. *Global Qualitative Nursing Research, 2*, 1–13. 10.1177/2333393615575313

Beck, C.T., Driscoll, J.W., & Watson, S. (2013). *Traumatic childbirth*. Routledge. 10.4324/9780203766699

Bergink, V., Gibney, S.M., & Drexhage, H.A. (2014). Autoimmunity, inflammation, and psychosis: A search for peripheral markers. *Biological Psychiatry, 75*(4), 324–331. 10.1016/j.biopsych.2013.09.037

Borrell-Carrió, F., Suchman, A.L., & Epstein, R.M. (2004). The biopsychosocial model 25 years later: Principles, practice, and scientific inquiry. *Annals of Family Medicine, 2*(6), 576–582. 10.1370/afm.245

Chen, M., & Lacey, R.E. (2018). Adverse childhood experiences and adult inflammation: Findings from the 1958 British Birth Cohort. *Brain, Behavior & Immunity, 69*, 582–590. 10.1016/j.bbi.2018.02.007

Danese, A., Moffitt, T.E., Harrington, H., Milne, B.J., Polanczyk, G., Pariante, C.M., & Caspi, A. (2009). Adverse childhood experiences and adult risk factors for age-related disease: Depression, inflammation, and clustering of metabolic risk factors. *Archives of Pediatric and Adolescent Medicine, 163*(12), 1135–1143. 10.1001/archpediatrics.2009.214

Duthie, L., & Reynolds, R.M. (2013). Changes in the maternal hypothalamic-pituitary-adrenal axis in pregnancy and postpartum: Influences on maternal and fetal outcomes. *Neuroendocrinology, 98*(2), 106–115. 10.1159/000354702

Finy, M.S., & Christian, L. (2018). Pathways linking childhood abuse history and current socioeconomic status to inflammation during pregnancy. *Brain, Behavior & Immunity, 74*, 231–240. 10.1016/j.bbi.2018.09.012

Ford, E., & Ayers, S. (2011). Support during birth interacts with prior trauma and birth intervention to predict postnatal post-traumatic stress symptoms. *Psychology & Health, 26*(12), 1553–1570. 10.1080/08870446.2010.533770

Gill, H., El-Halabi, S., Majeed, A., Gill, B., Lui, L.M.W., Mansur, R.B., ... Rosenblat, J.D. (2020). The association between Adverse Childhood Experiences and inflammation in patients with major depressive disorder: A systematic review. *Journal of Affective Disorders, 272*, 1–7. 0.1016/j.jad.2020.03.145

Grisbrook, M.A., & Letourneau, N. (2021). Improving maternal postpartum mental health screening guidelines requires assessment of post-traumatic stress disorder. *Canadian Journal of Public Health, 112*(2), 240–243. 10.17269/s41997-020-00373-8

Hill, D. (2015). *Affect regulation theory. A clinical model.* Norton.

Iyengar, U., Rajhans, R., Fonagy, P., Strathearn, L., & Kim, S. (2019). Unresolved trauma and reorganization in mothers: Attachment and neuroscience perspectives. *Frontiers in Psychology, 10*, 110. 10.3389/fpsyg.2019.00110

Kendall-Tackett, K.A. (2007). A new paradigm for depression in new mothers: The central role of inflammation and how breastfeeding and anti-inflammatory treatments protect maternal mental health. *International Breastfeeding Journal, 2*(6). 10.1186/1746-4358-2-6

Kendall-Tackett, K.A. (2010). Four research findings that will change what we think about perinatal depression. *The Journal of Perinatal Education, 19*(4), 7–9. 10.1624/105812410X530875

Kendall-Tackett, K.A. (2017a). *Depression in new mothers. Causes, consequences, and treatment alternatives.* 3rd ed. Routledge.

Kendall-Tackett, K.A. (2017b). Why trauma-informed care needs to be the standard of care for IBCLCs. Editorial. *Clinical Lactation, 8*(4), 150–151. 10.1891/2158-0782.8.4.150

Kendall-Tackett, K.A. (2019). Creating an oxytocic environment for new mothers. Editorial. *Clinical Lactation, 10*(1), 7–8. 10.1891/2158-0782.10.1.7

Kendall-Tackett, K.A., & Beck, C.T. (2022). Secondary traumatic stress and moral injury in maternity care providers: A narrative and exploratory review. *Frontiers in Global Women's Health, 3*. 10.3389/fgwh.2022/835811

Kendall-Tackett, K.A., Cong, Z., & Hale, T.W. (2015). Birth interventions related to lower rates of exclusive breastfeeding and increased risk of postpartum depression in a large sample. *Clinical Lactation, 6*(3), 87–97. 10.1891/2158-0782.6.3.87

Kim, S., & Strathearn, L. (2016). Oxytocin and maternal brain plasticity. *New Directions for Child and Adolescent Development, 2016*(153), 59–72. 10.1002/cad.20170

Kingston, D., & Mughal, M.K. (2020). Overview of perinatal maternal stress. In R.M. Quatraro & P. Grussu (Eds.), *Handbook of perinatal clinical psychology. From theory to practice* (pp. 8–25). Routledge. 10.4324/9780429351990

Lee, C.H., & Giuliani, F. (2019) The role of inflammation in depression and fatigue. *Frontiers in Immunology, 10*, 1696. 10.3389/fimmu.2019.01696

Levine, P.A. (2010). *In an unspoken voice. How the body releases trauma and restores goodness.* North Atlantic Books.

Padin, A.C., Stevens, N.R., Che, M.L., Erondu, I.N., Perera, M.J., & Shalowitz, M.U. (2022). Screening for PTSD during pregnancy: A missed opportunity. *BMC Pregnancy and Childbirth, 22*(1), 487. 10.1186/s12884-022-04797-7

Pawluski, J.L., Lonstein, J.S., & Fleming, A.S. (2017). The neurobiology of postpartum anxiety and depression. *Trends in Neurosciences, 40*(2), 106–120. 10.1016/j.tins.2016.11.009

Quinones, M.M., Gallegos, A.M., Lin, F.V., & Heffner, K. (2020). Dysregulation of inflammation, neurobiology, and cognitive function in PTSD: An integrative review. *Cognitive, Affective, & Behavioral Neuroscience, 20*, 455–480. 10.3758/s13415-020-00782-9

Seng, J.S., Low, L.K., Sperlich, M., Ronis, D.L., & Liberzon, I. (2009). Prevalence, trauma history, and risk for posttraumatic stress disorder among nulliparous women in maternity care. *Obstetrics & Gynecology, 114*(4), 839–847. 10.1097/AOG.0b013e3181b8f8a2

Uchino, B.N., Trettevik, R., Kent de Grey, R.G., Cronan, S., Hogan, J., & Baucom, B.R.W. (2018). Social support, social integration, and inflammatory cytokines: A meta-analysis. *Health Psychology, 37*(5), 462–471. 10.1037/hea0000594

Uvnäs-Moberg, K. (2014). *Oxytocin: The biological guide to motherhood.* Praeclarus Press.

Venta, A., Bick, J., & Bechelli, J. (2021). COVID-19 threatens maternal mental health and infant development: Possible paths from stress and isolation to adverse outcomes and a call for research and practice. *Child Psychiatry & Human Development, 52*, 200–204. 10.1007/s10578-021-01140-7

3
Resisting Patriarchal Motherhood
From Maternal Bodylessness to Maternal Bodyfulness

The Institution of Motherhood and the Emergence of Matricentric Feminism

Although the question of the maternal has a conflictual history of being marginalized in the field of feminism (O'Reilly, 2021), motherhood is crucial for analyzing the oppression of women (Bueskens, 2018). Motherhood has been identified as "the unfinished business of feminism" (O'Reilly, 2019, p. 13). In 1976 in her landmark book *Of Women Born*, Rich introduced the distinction between a woman's personal potential for mothering and the institution of motherhood that aims to keep women and their reproductive potential under male control. This distinction marked a significant shift in feminist thinking about mothering and how mothers are impacted by patriarchal structures and inaugurated the field of maternal theory, which has become a distinct academic discipline over the last three decades (O'Reilly, 2019, 2020). Rich (1976) critically analyzed how motherhood functions in a patriarchal culture and thereby inspired a new school of feminist thinking and research centering on mothers that up until then had been absent in feminist scholarship. The field of maternal theory was formulated by O'Reilly (2007, 2020) and builds on Rich's distinction between "motherhood as institution and ideology, and mothering as experience and identity" (O'Reilly, 2020, p. 19). The distinction introduced by Rich was monumental firstly because it pawed the way for a new critical analysis of how patriarchy oppresses women in particular ways through the institution of motherhood, and secondly, because it inspired a new envisioning of mothering as a potentially empowering way to resist this oppression. O'Reilly's (2021) rationale for feminism focusing on mothers is that mothers face distinct forms of social, economic, political, cultural, and psychological problems related to their identity as mothers and how it is perceived by the patriarchal institution of motherhood. Matricentric feminism is built on the recognition of a need for a distinctive feminism for and about mothers and a distinction between the categories of mother and woman (O'Reilly, 2020).

The movements of matricentric feminism and feminist mothering were born from maternal theory scholarship and assume that mothering can be a site of empowerment and social change if mothers are freed from the oppressive dynamics of patriarchal motherhood (Green, 2004; O'Reilly, 2020). Another important concept that fueled the emergence of maternal theory is Ruddick's (1989) work on maternal practice and maternal thinking, introducing a new way of understanding mothering as an individual, lived, reflective, and skillful practice as opposed to an instinctual habit that fulfills a prescriptive and normative role. Matricentric feminism understands the term "mother" broadly as anyone engaging in motherwork (O'Reilly, 2019), or what Ruddick (1989) called maternal practice. From this focus, mothering is also understood more as a practice than as an identity (O'Reilly, 2019). In matricentric feminist thinking, the focus of critical analysis is not only on patriarchy in general but specifically on the institution of patriarchal motherhood. It explores mothers' particular needs, experiences, and desires and the ways mothers are oppressed in a patriarchal culture.

In matricentric feminism, mothering is repositioned from the private to the political dimension: The practices of mothering, or maternal practice (Ruddick, 1989), are seen as a socially and politically meaningful engaged practice. The core belief is that maternal agency and activism lead to social and political change: "[M]otherwork for feminist mothers is a transformative practice in that it both embodies and instructs upon the possibilities of and for social and political change" (O'Reilly, 2007, p. 172). A central tenet of matricentric feminism is that patriarchal motherhood is culturally and socially constructed and can therefore be challenged as such (O'Reilly, 2020), making it highly relevant for a biopsychosocial understanding of the maternal transition. Social dynamics, cultural expectations, and systemic inequalities have been established as central factors in Maternal Mental Health, making the question of social change pressing for mothering and mothers' conditions and especially their mental health. O'Reilly (2020) has argued that the discourses on normative motherhood are responses to and results of cultural and economic changes. This recognition of the political dimensions of mothering is central to matricentric feminism. The fields of maternal theory and matricentric feminism have evolved with critical analyses of societal discourses and narratives related to the institution of motherhood and how they affect women and mothers. A key concept for this development is the term "intensive mothering" introduced by Hays (1996), who studied the cultural contradictions of motherhood.

Intensive Mothering and the Dictates of Patriarchal Motherhood

Hays (1996) argued that the values of family life, and mothering in particular, contradict the values of economic and political life. She described the cultural ideals of mothering as an ideology of "intensive mothering" characterized by three tenets: That mothers are inherently better parents than fathers, that mothering should be child-centered, and that children are inherently fulfilling to mothers. Hays' data analysis revealed that both traditional stay-at-home mothers and working mothers are faced with the cultural contradictions of motherhood; both groups rely on the assumptions of the intensive mothering ideology when coping with ambivalence and worries about their parenting. Paradoxically, both groups seek explanations for contradicting cultural values that can confirm the rightness of their choices. Hays (1996) also pointed out the paradox that ideals for mothering and motherhood culture have become increasingly intensive and demanding as women have expanded their role in the workforce. Bueskens (2018; 2019) contends that it is indeed this shift in late modernity of women into the workforce and a position of legal equality that is causing a paradox: Women are freer as individuals in modern society, but they remain constrained through motherhood. Women face significant economic challenges from taking time for maternity leave as well as combining paid and unpaid work as working mothers (Bueskens, 2019). The freedoms women have gained in modern society relate directly to the difficulties they experience as mothers (Bueskens, 2018, 2019). Bueskens' theory on the paradox of women's dual roles in late modern society captures the tensions of mothering from the contradictory place of being a legal free subject while simultaneously having that freedom restricted by one's position as a mother, as the position of the free individual impinges on the maternal position by being defined by its differentiation from it, aligned with Stone's (2014) analysis. The intensive mothering ideology must be understood in this historical context of women's changed rights and roles in a Western post-industrialized world.

O'Reilly (2020) contends that while there are precursors to the current form of intensive mothering ideology in the post-war period, it did not emerge fully until the late 1980s and 1990s due to a number of reasons, including demographic changes, class dynamics, and the rise of widely available knowledge from developmental psychology and child research. The development of the intensive mothering ideology must also be examined in the context of the mid-1990s' developments of consumerism and politically driven neoliberal restrictions of social and financial support for families (Ennis, 2014). Hays

(1996) pointed out the contradiction of mothers being expected to engage in "unselfish nurturing" in a society that is influenced by consumerism's strong focus on the individual and understanding of self-interest as a main driver of behavior.

The ideals of patriarchal motherhood and intensive mothering are oppressive through the social pressure on women to conform to the cultural expectations for good mothering (Green, 2019). Scholars have continued Hays' work with critical analysis of contemporary developments of intensive mothering ideology. O'Reilly (2021) has expanded on the concept of intensive mothering with her theory on how patriarchal motherhood is oppressive to women through several ideological assumptions and dictates about what normative motherhood is. O'Reilly (2021) has identified no less than ten dictates of normative motherhood: Essentialization (that all women want to be mothers), privatization (that mothering is done in the private sphere), individualization (that mothering is done by one person), naturalization (that mothering abilities are innate), normalization (that mothering is done in the context of the nuclear family), idealization (that all mothers find joy and fulfillment in motherhood), biologicalization (that biological mothers are more authentic mothers), expertization (that mothering must be guided by experts), intensification (that mothering must be intense and time-consuming), and depoliticalization (that mothering is private and non-political). Through these dictates, patriarchal motherhood and intensive mothering ideology isolate mothers because it stipulates that mothers must raise their children in isolation in the private realm, primarily alone as the sole caregiver, as an activity outside the realm of democracy, and that it is time-consuming and intense (O'Reilly, 2021). Mothers who cannot or will not live up to these dictates experience othering dynamics of being positioned as bad mothers (O'Reilly, 2021). Examples of some activities that intensive mothering include are mothers' social lives revolving around their children, mothers spending all their free time with their children, or mothers putting their children's needs before their own (Ennis, 2014). The intensification lies in the mother's investment of much, if not all, of her "time, labor, emotion, intellect, and money in their children" (Hays, 1996, p. 130).

Matricentric Feminism and Feminist Psychoanalysis

Matricentric feminism is interdisciplinary and draws on related fields of study like feminist psychoanalysis (O'Reilly, 2019). O'Reilly (2021) has emphasized how patriarchal motherhood is deeply oppressive to women because the woman's selfhood is denied or repressed by its demands and dictates. In this way, matricentric feminism presents a sociological analysis of the issues of maternal subjectivity that feminist intersubjective psychoanalysis analyzes psychologically. Where feminist psychoanalysis understands the issues of the erasure of maternal subjectivity as a result of how subjectivity in modern Western culture is structured in opposition to the maternal body (Stone, 2014), matricentric feminism illuminates how the patriarchal institution of motherhood works on a societal level to oppress mothers by defining and governing their maternal status through dictates and norms that undermine their individual expression and experience of mothering as a lived practice. Feminist psychoanalysis and matricentric feminism align and complement each other in their critical analyses and attention to the question of maternal subjectivity from different levels of analysis. Furthermore, they share a focus on valuing the perspective and voice of the mother, a "matrifocial" perspective (O'Reilly, 2019).

Feminist psychoanalysis has acknowledged the conflictual role of cultural prescriptive and normative ideals of mothering like those of intensive mothering (Parker, 1995), and has critically examined the consequences of idealizations of motherhood (Benjamin, 1988, 1994). Based on her qualitative research and re-reading of classic psychoanalysis from a matrifocal perspective, Parker (1995) concluded that mothers often experience dissonance and tension between their subjective experiences of mothering and the normative ideals of motherhood. This makes it hard for mothers to negotiate their lived experience with the cultural expectations for mothering, which is important for processing maternal ambivalence (Parker, 1995). The child-centric focus of intensive mothering and normative motherhood is in direct opposition to intersubjective feminist psychoanalysis' understanding of the developmental function and necessity of differentiated maternal subjectivity. Idealization of the mother undermines her subjectivity and positions separation (both physical separation through absence and figurative separation as differentiation and disagreement) as inherently problematic (Benjamin, 1988). Feminist psychoanalysis contributes to matricentric feminism with a critical analysis of intensive mothering ideology through a critique of the way its idealization of mothers undermines maternal subjectivity (Vissing, 2014).

The cultural discourse on intensive mothering is particularly problematic for maternal subjectivity because of the way it positions motherhood as an essentialized measure of objective truth, at the expense of the subjective experience of mothering. I have previously argued that a key problem with discourses on the "rightness" of different mothering styles is that the debates happen at the expense of acknowledging individual maternal subjectivity: Mothers' experiences become underpinnings or "tales of proof" for a parenting philosophy in the belligerent debates and are thus lost as voices in their own rights (Vissing, 2014). Intensive mothering ideology operates with an unrealistic understanding of mothers and their mothering which idealizes their presence and demonizes their absence and ambivalence. This stifles the individual mother's potential for asserting her maternal subjectivity and processing her ambivalence (Vissing, 2014). This is a psychosocial dynamic of the problem with maternal subjectivity and a symptom of the continued pervasiveness of the intensive mothering ideology. Matricentric feminism is an important contribution to feminist psychoanalysis and biopsychosocial thinking because it is a useful analytic tool for reckoning with the psychosocial dynamics in Maternal Mental Health.

How Intensive Mothering Ideology Affects Maternal Mental Health

As reviewed above, matricentric feminist analyses have critiqued societal discourse and narratives of "good mothering" for producing unrealistically high expectations for mothers

(Ennis, 2014; Hays, 1996; Warner, 2005). But beyond theoretical critique and analyses, researchers have also done quantitative and qualitative studies that demonstrate connections between the guilt and shame associated with not meeting these unrealistic standards for mothering and increased symptoms of stress, depression, and anxiety (Henderson et al., 2016; Liss et al., 2012; Meeussen & Van Laar, 2018; Rizzo et al., 2012; Sockol et al., 2014). Rizzo et al. (2012) studied the connections between parents' attitudes about parenting and their mental health outcomes, specifically how intensive mothering beliefs correlate with mental health. Their research demonstrated that intensive mothering beliefs indeed correlate with several negative mental health outcomes, and the results made the researchers conclude that negative maternal mental health outcomes may be accounted for by the endorsement of intensive parenting attitudes. However, research has also indicated that the pressures to live up to the high standards of intensive mothering are related to increased guilt and stress *even when the mothers do not hold strong beliefs of intensive mothering* (Henderson et al., 2016). This could be related to mothers' fears of the social penalties of failing to meet the high standards of intensive mothering as indicated by research by Liss et al. (2012), also reflected in O'Reilly's (2021) theory on the dictates of normative motherhood and the consequences of not living up to them. A systemic review of qualitative studies demonstrated unrealistic expectations as a common theme for mothers (McCarthy et al., 2021). Across studies, women reported anxiety and stress due to pressure to adhere to perceived social expectations and ideas about motherhood. Additionally, the stigma associated with PMADs was identified as a theme and a barrier to seeking help in several studies. One study indicated that mothers may feel that being overwhelmed in the postpartum period is indicative of "failure", creating barriers to their help-seeking (Bilszta et al., 2010).

Despite the pressure of the cultural expectations for mothers, Meeussen and Van Laar (2018) point out that mothers are not passive recipients of intensive mothering norms but actively try to regulate and negotiate this pressure. While mothers may be oppressed and harmed by intensive mothering ideology, Ennis (2014) has pointed out that behaviors that persist must also serve an underlying purpose. I have suggested a feminist psychoanalytic theory (Vissing, 2014) on the protective functions of the idealization of the mother that is prevalent in intensive mothering ideology. Based on Parker's (1995) understanding of maternal ambivalence as crucial for maternal development and Benjamin's (1988, 1995) theory of maternal subjectivity as the foundation for the development of intersubjective capacities, I argue that the idea of the perfect mother in intensive mothering is reflective of a fantasy that protects against the anxieties related to maternal ambivalence and maternal differentiation (Vissing, 2014). The experiences of maternal ambivalence and asserting maternal subjectivity are inherently conflictual and anxiety-producing and must therefore be processed, reflected on, and integrated in a developmental sense. A cultural discourse on motherhood like intensive mothering that 1. does not allow for much openness about maternal ambivalence and 2. understands a mother's differentiation and needs for her own space, physically and figuratively, as inherently wrong, makes it very hard for any mother to process her ambivalence and assert her subjectivity by navigating her lived experience of mothering with the cultural expectations put on her. Intensive mothering ideology offers the idea that it is possible to be a perfect mother by living up to certain standards. In this way, endorsing intensive mothering beliefs may offer protection against anxieties about one's limitations for and ambivalence about mothering. Personal self-protection against anxieties is embedded in culturally conveyed dictates of institutionalized motherhood.

It is well-documented that disparities in Maternal Mental Health are related to sociodemographic and cultural diversity (see Introduction to Part I). Matricentric feminism is informed by intersectional analysis (O'Reilly, 2019), which is key to understanding disparities in Maternal Mental Health. Matricentric feminism builds on an underlying understanding that the institution of motherhood affects mothers differently depending on socioeconomic and cultural factors like age, class, ethnicity, race, and sexual orientation (Green, 2019; O'Reilly, 2020). The demands of the cultural expectations for mothers, especially unrealistically high standards, must be understood from this intersectional perspective. Garland McKinney and Meinersmann (2022) have pointed out that while the demands of motherhood alone may contribute to Mental Health issues, the intersection of the maternal role with other markers of identity like race, ethnicity, gender identity, sexual orientation, or socioeconomic status present unique circumstances. Ennis (2014) has pointed out that contexts of undoing of public support and welfare resources make it even harder to meet the standards for intensive mothering, disproportionately impacting mothers of lower socio-economic status.

Feminist and Empowered Mothering

While motherhood as a patriarchal institution restricts and oppresses mothers through the dictates of normative motherhood, the subjective experience of mothering can be empowering and a way to resist the oppression of patriarchal motherhood (Green, 2019; O'Reilly, 2021). It is this assumption that inspired the movement of feminist mothering (Green, 2019). Indeed, it is this distinction of the reality of patriarchal mothering that makes feminist mothering possible (O'Reilly, 2019). Feminist mothering can be understood as the lived praxis of matricentric feminism (Green, 2004, 2019). Green (2019) describes feminist mothering as "the process of joining one's feminism together with one's parenting" (p. 83). The primary aim of feminist mothering is the empowerment of mothers through resistance against patriarchal motherhood. O'Reilly (2007) defines feminist mothering as "any practice of mothering that seeks to challenge and change various aspects of patriarchal motherhood that cause mothering to be limiting or oppressive to women" (p. 168).

It is a key belief in feminist mothering that mothering *can* be a site of empowerment (Green, 2004), which is a view that some second-wave feminists do not share (O'Reilly, 2020). Green

(2004) contended that it is in a mother's nurturing of her growth through her mothering and her relationship with her child that she actively undermines institutionalized motherhood and challenges patriarchal structures. Feminist mothering emphasizes that mothers continue their development as full individuals with self-hood "outside and beyond motherhood" (O'Reilly, 2021, p. 167). In this way, feminist mothering is a way of disrupting the child-centric model of mothering that is prevalent in intensive mothering and challenging the hegemonic ideals of the good mother (Green, 2019). Through the practice of feminist mothering, matricentric feminism thus expands maternal subjectivity while refusing the notions that motherhood is inherently only oppressive to women and that women's identities are defined solely by it. Through qualitative research with self-identified feminist mothers, Green (2009) observed that when the mothers identified and critically reflected on the ways they experienced the institution of motherhood as oppressive, they engaged in self-reflection about their maternal subjectivity that empowered them to redefine motherhood for themselves. Before the movement of feminist mothering became visible, parenting was not seen as part of organized feminist activism (Green, 2019). In Green's (2019) interviews with feminist mothers, she found that they understood their daily activities of mothering as a feminist praxis for directly creating social change.

O'Reilly (2021) distinguishes between feminist and empowered mothering to acknowledge that some mothers who do not identify as feminists engage in empowering mothering practices. Feminist mothering is done by mothers who understand their feminism "as an embodied identity" and see their feminist activism and mothering as intertwined (Green, 2019, p. 87). Empowered mothering encompasses all forms of mothering that empower mothers to resist patriarchal motherhood. Feminist mothering thus refers to a particular kind of empowered mothering based on feminist identification (O'Reilly, 2021). While there is significant overlap between the two, O'Reilly (2021) notes the importance of distinguishing between them because women may have different reasons for choosing to mother in ways that go against the normative expectations of patriarchal motherhood. Feminist mothers understand their mothering choices as intertwined with their feminist activism, where empowered mothers make choices for mothering for personal reasons that they don't necessarily connect to any political activism. From a clinical perspective, this distinction is important to avoid making assumptions about mothers' ways of mothering and their underlying political beliefs and refrain from imposing expectations for feminist beliefs on mothers. The concept of empowered mothering is crucial to Maternal Mental Health because it acknowledges that mothers' personal choices for how to mother can be a way to actively resist oppressive cultural expectations for motherhood that are related to poor mental health.

O'Reilly (2007) identified five central tenets of empowered mothering: Agency, autonomy, authenticity, authority, and advocacy/activism. Empowered mothering is formed on the understanding of mothering as carrying significance and purpose, which stands in contrast to the notions of mothering as private and apolitical in patriarchal motherhood (O'Reilly, 2021). O'Reilly (2021) points out that empowered mothering recognizes that both mother and child benefit when the mother has agency, authority, authenticity, and autonomy in her life and mothering. Examples of empowering mothering practices are focusing on the importance of mothers' needs being met, acknowledging that mothering does not fulfill all of a woman's needs, not believing that mothers are solely responsible for how children turn out, and challenging mainstream parenting practices (O'Reilly, 2021). In this way, empowered mothering is a way to counter the narratives of intensive mothering ideology by actively questioning societal expectations for mothers, especially what a "good" mother is, and asserting one's own beliefs and preferences for mothering. Empowered mothering is about questioning the expectations of intensive mothering ideology and patriarchal motherhood, in all thinkable ways, from a place of personal agency. This includes the ways patriarchal motherhood impacts mothers' bodies and their embodied sense of self.

Somatic Consequences of Patriarchal Motherhood: Maternal Bodylessness

Caldwell (2018a, 2018b) has analyzed and described the underlying dynamics of the individual and societal phenomenon of the marginalization of the body, captured with the term bodylessness. There are four overlapping aspects of bodylessness: Ignoring the body, seeing the body as an object or project, hating the body (somatophobia), and making one's own or other's bodies wrong (somaticism) (Caldwell, 2018a). Bodylessness is thus caused by ignoring, objectifying, devaluing, or shunning certain bodies. The harm of these actions lies in the way they disrupt a person's sense of body identity. Laing (2021) has suggested that all forms of prejudice are driven by "horror of the body itself" and a displacement of this fear onto other bodies (p. 272). Bodylessness manifests concretely as self-regulation issues, a lack of sensory awareness, and as a lack of embodied sense of self where bodily experiences are integrated and made sense of as part of one's identity and lived experience. Leighton (2018) has pointed out that devaluing the body (somatophobia) is a kind of trauma in itself. Systemic oppression and discrimination are concrete experiences felt in the body and can happen in subtle and insidious ways, with severe consequences for one's health and well-being (Caldwell, 2018b).

Bodylessness in relation to the maternal body relates to the lack of recognition of embodied maternal subjectivity. The four aspects of bodylessness manifest in the perinatal context in several ways listed in Table 3.1. The othering dynamics towards mothers that come from the problem of not recognizing maternal subjectivity result in objectification of the maternal body. The bodily aspects of the maternal experience are ignored or minimized when the maternal body is medicalized and understudied. For example, there is a significant gap in medical research on pregnant women (Little & Wickremsinhe, 2017). Furthermore, patriarchal motherhood disconnects subjectivity from maternal embodiment through the dictates of normative motherhood that implies an arbitrary standard of the maternal identity built on ideological values. In patriarchal motherhood, the maternal body becomes a means to fulfill the dictates and expectations of a societal role, as opposed to the corporeal individuality of the mother as a full person whose mothering and subjectivity are mutually constitutive through her embodiment. From a matricentric feminist perspective, the oppressive dynamics of bodylessness in society impact mothers in these ways that are different from the forms of bodylessness experienced by non-mothers.

O'Brien Hallstein (2015) has expanded the understanding of intensive mothering in her analysis of how bodily standards for mothers are intensified through celebrity culture. She argues that contemporary feminine and maternal identity is connected to the neoliberal understanding of the body and what she calls "body work" in relation to gender. This is a way of making the body a project, for example through intense pressures for healthy body management and idealization of a quick return to the pre-pregnancy body, mediated through celebrity culture, adding a dimension of class. In this way, contemporary intensive mothering ideology has evolved to include a focus on the body as a site of the unrealistic standards of mothering. The notion that a mother's body can appear seemingly "untouched" by having given birth as a positive outcome is reflective of somatophobia in that it builds on an assumption that the bodily consequences of giving birth are inherently negative, effectively imbuing all maternal bodies with wrongness. In other words, patriarchal motherhood turns women into bodies that birth instead of full subjects who have their identity transformed in a developmental and embodied sense by becoming mothers. It is namely through the paradoxical combination of ignoring of the maternal body and the somatophobia and somaticism towards it that mothers' embodied subjectivity is undermined. Disconnecting subjectivity from embodiment is a dehumanizing form of oppression, as it causes a person to be reduced to flesh and bodies to be seen as materials devoid of personhood. The dictates of patriarchal motherhood land on the maternal body as patterns of profound over-exertion, dysregulation, and bodylessness.

TABLE 3.1 Aspects of Maternal Bodylessness

Ignoring the body	Stigma and shame related to the maternal body and perinatal body experiences Minimizing perinatal sensations Lack of research involving pregnant women
Seeing the body as object or project	Medicalizing the maternal body Erasing maternal subjectivity from maternal embodiment Unrealistic expectations for mothering and the maternal body Weaponizing of the maternal body in politics
Hating the body (somatophobia)	Disconnecting emotional aspects from medical aspects of the maternal transition Shame and privatizing related to the postpartum body Idealizing bodies that are "untouched" by the maternal transition
Making bodies wrong (somaticism)	Othering non-normative maternal/perinatal bodies Narratives of "failures" of the maternal body

Body Identity and Bodyfulness

In contrast to the concept of bodylessness, the concepts of body identity and bodyfulness expand and enrich the understanding of the embodied sense of self. The concept of body identity builds on assumption from narrative identity theory that the body self is expressed and narrated through nonverbal communication (Caldwell, 2016). The understanding is that when untold narratives of the self are told, identity is formed. This aligns with the psychoanalytic principle that continuous processing of unconscious material is necessary to conscious integration of a person's self-state. Caldwell (2016) contends that when we combine nonverbal and verbal storytelling in self-narratives, our concept of identity is enriched and extended by including the embodied aspects of self. Caldwell's (2018a) concept of bodyfulness includes both practices of sensory awareness and a reflective attitude towards one's body narrative and body identity that manifests as responsiveness to bodily experiences. Bodyfulness is thus more than awareness of sensations. It involves the somatic listening skills of sensory awareness, but also responsive connectedness to one's body and reflexivity about one's body identity (2018a, 2018b). In a sense, the body becomes an interlocutor for the ongoing discovery of one's sense of self.

Caldwell (2018a) states that bodyfulness is about holding the embodied self in a "conscious, contemplative environment" (p. xxiii). This facilitates a reclaiming of oneself through the body and bodily focused contemplation. Bodyfulness is therefore aimed at cultivating a sense of self and agency through the integration of experiential knowledge and nonverbal body narratives. Through bodyfulness, the body is appreciated as the foundation of identity (2018a) and a potential site of resistance (2018b). Caldwell (2018a) contends that in a culture that marginalizes the body and bodily experiences, even using the word bodyful can hold political meaning. The philosophy of bodyfulness is that knowing oneself is a process of experiencing, responding to, and reflecting on - *and with* - the body. This includes the layers of identity that are politically salient, like maternal identity.

Bodyfulness is relevant to the maternal transition in several ways. The development that the new mother self undergoes originates in a bodily transformation and the way it reorganizes her subjectivity. The root of her new maternal self must therefore be found in the new maternal body experiences and narratives that are the basis of the emerging maternal body self. Experiencing the new maternal body is a sensory experience, but it must then be integrated and made sense of through responsiveness towards and reflection on these new sensations, which is the essence of bodyfulness. The new maternal self-narrative is formed from both bodily experiences and reflective processing of them. This processing does not have to be completely verbalized, as it is in the interplay between the non-verbal and the verbal that new meanings of being an embodied maternal subject emerge. Caldwell (2018a) points out that it is namely the connection between nonverbal body expressions and our verbalized expressions that give our words meaning. Nonverbal narratives expressed with and through the body and verbalized self-narratives are mutually constitutive and synergistically related. This dynamic holds a unique potential for empowerment in relation to the maternal transition as it is characterized by being a bodily transformation that reorganizes subjectivity and thrusts the mother into a realm of nonverbal coregulatory relating, all of which happens under challenging circumstances of internal anxieties and external cultural pressures. By claiming the body as the site of assertion of subjectivity, a mother can circumvent the erasure of her subjectivity and the bodylessness caused by patriarchal motherhood.

Maternal Bodyfulness as Empowered Mothering

Empowered or feminist mothering can take many forms and is not formulaic or dictated by any authority (Green, 2019). It is defined by the way it empowers mothers to fight against the oppression that patriarchal motherhood causes. From the understanding that patriarchal motherhood causes maternal bodylessness, healing of perinatal trauma as an embodied relational process becomes a form of resistance against the patriarchal narrative of motherhood and thus an empowered mothering practice. Mothers' healing of trauma is understood in a wider biopsychosocial context when it is connected to the psychosocial dynamics of patriarchal oppressive structures. Caldwell (2018a) states that just as oppression and marginalization are experienced through the body, activism is enacted through and within the body. In the same vein, Laing (2021) argues that the body can be a force of freedom in its own right and thus a tool for resistance. When feminist or empowered mothering practices are connected to the concept of bodyfulness and focused on embodied assertion of maternal subjectivity, they become ways of challenging somatophobia and somaticism against the maternal body and claiming and recovering maternal body identity.

Maternal bodyfulness is bodily focused resistance against the dictates of patriarchal motherhood by actively challenging the oppression of the maternal body. It is based on the integration of the assumption of feminist mothering that mothering can be a site of empowerment (Green, 2004; O'Reilly, 2020) and the assumption of somatic psychology that bodies can be a resource of resistance (Caldwell & Leighton, 2018). Feminist mothering is about reclaiming power and agency. When mothers define and claim their mothering and maternal subjectivity for themselves, it becomes a creative assertion of self (Green, 2009). Caldwell's (2018b) somatic approach describes political activism as inherently somatic in that our embodiment and expression of body narrative and body identity cannot be separated from political life. Claiming our body self is therefore a crucial way to claim agency. When we integrate this somatic approach with the values of feminist mothering, we see the potential for working somatically with mothers. Somatic interventions in the perinatal period are potent for individual trauma healing and self-regulation and for political activism through claiming embodied agency and authority of self. From this feminist somatic approach, the perinatal trauma healing process involves a replacement of maternal bodylessness with maternal bodyfulness. In this process, maternal bodyfulness is the development of a deeper experiential knowledge of one's subjectivity as a mother. This is more than sensory awareness; it is about developing an embodied and reflective relationship to one's new maternal identity where one's mothering is discovered as an expression of self as opposed to a role prescribed by cultural expectations. Based on a bottom-up perspective of appreciating body experiences and narratives as the foundation for any sense of self, it is a vision of asserting oneself as a maternal subject through and with the body.

From this foundation, maternal bodyfulness is a feminist and somatic practice aimed at preventing and circumventing the effects of maternal bodylessness. It is the concretization of asserting maternal subjectivity. This philosophy of maternal bodyfulness aligns with the understanding of "feminism as an embodied identity" (Green, 2019, p. 87). Concretely, maternal bodyfulness is the therapeutic work that supports mothers in claiming their maternal embodied subjectivity by cultivating their agency and autonomy through sensory awareness skills and self-regulation practices that relate *and are specific to* the maternal transition and identity. This situates the mother as the authority of her developing maternal self through her somatic and emotional transformation and is thereby a form of resisting patriarchal motherhood and intensive mothering ideology. Minimizing and erasing the embodied aspects of the perinatal transition are countered by cultivating maternal sensory awareness. The five tenets of empowered mothering (agency, autonomy, authenticity, authority, and advocacy/activism) (O'Reilly, 2021) align with the somatic concepts of bodyfulness and body identity (Caldwell, 2016, 2018a) and are central to building maternal sensory awareness skills. Maternal bodyfulness is based on the mother being the authority of the bodily experience of her maternal transition meaning only she can define what it means for her to have and be a maternal body and to mother in an embodied sense. The therapeutic approach must therefore be one of centering the mother's somatic experiences by supporting her discovery and awareness of them and her agency in navigating and regulating them.

Maternal bodyfulness must be understood as both verbal and nonverbal practices. As maternal subjectivity originates in preverbal bodily differentiation, it cannot be meaningfully asserted or identified as a purely mental concept. It must be experienced both as nonverbal embodied expressions of self and verbal body narratives of those experiences. The concept of maternal bodyfulness offers a counter-narrative of mothering in opposition to the disembodied dictates of normative motherhood, but this is a narrative that may or may not be fully verbalized. On a psychosocial and activism level, a somatically focused approach to healing perinatal trauma offers mothers a vision for an empowered mode of mothering that resists the institution of patriarchal motherhood. This vision may be verbally explored in the therapeutic process, but it may also take nonverbal forms of co- or self-regulatory shifts. Language that is expanded by a sensory awareness vocabulary and assertion of maternal subjectivity can be cultivated in the therapeutic space to empower expecting and new mothers to formulate their own potential for mothering and assert their maternal subjectivity. Therapeutic ways of working towards maternal bodyfulness with sensory awareness and vocabulary will be presented in Chapter 6. The goal of such language building is not to verbalize all aspects of a mother's maternal body narrative and body identity, but to support her agency and authority in her journey of consciously discovering and *experiencing* her embodied sense of her maternal self.

Matricentric Feminist Mothering, Somatic Psychology, and Perinatal Trauma-Healing

In matricentric feminism, individual autonomy and choice are highly valued (Green, 2019; O'Reilly, 2021). The five tenets of matricentric feminism, agency, autonomy, authenticity, authority, and advocacy/activism, align with principles of trauma-informed care. Especially the principles of collaboration and mutuality, empowerment, voice, and choice, and historical, cultural, racial, ethnic, gender, and diversity issues (see Table 0.1 in Introduction to Part I). In matricentric feminism, motherhood is seen as both the site of oppression and the potential empowerment of mothers. Similarly, in trauma-informed somatic psychology, the body is understood as both the site of responses to trauma and the site of trauma healing and reclaiming of self through bodyfulness. Leighton (2018) has pointed out that there is a somatic cost to both colluding with and fighting back against oppression: It wears on the individual on a physical level. Similarly, Laing (2021) has pointed out how politics can turn bodies into prisons through prejudice and oppression, but that political transformation also happens from bodily activism. This struggle is acknowledged in feminist mothering philosophy that understands mothering as a site of both oppression and possibilities for empowerment. Green (2019) also describes feminist mothering as "embodied knowledge". From a trauma-informed perspective, healing and recovery is a process that goes beyond symptom reduction and involves an understanding of the healing process as a developmental struggle towards agency and autonomy. Feminist or empowered mothering practices align with these principles of trauma-informed care and bring them into a political and societal context.

References

Benjamin, J. (1988). *The bonds of love: Psychoanalysis, feminism, and the problem of domination*. Pantheon Books.

Benjamin, J. (1994). The omnipotent mother: A psychoanalytic study of fantasy and reality. In D. Bassin, M. Honey, & M.M. Kaplan (Eds.), *Representations of motherhood* (pp. 129–147). Yale University Press.

Benjamin, J. (1995). *Like subjects, loveobjects: Essays on recognition and sexual difference*. University Press.

Bilszta, J.L., Ericksen, J., Buist, A.E., & Milgrom, J. (2010). Women's experience of postnatal depression – Beliefs and attitudes as barriers to care. *The Australian Journal of Advanced Nursing, 27*(3), 44–54.

Bueskens, P. (2018). *Modern motherhood and women's dual identities: Rewriting the sexual contract*. Routledge. 10.4324/9781315559520

Bueskens, P. (2019). Deregulated patriarchy and the new sexual contract: One step forward and two steps back. *Journal of the Motherhood Initiative for Research and Community Involvement, 10*(1/2), 59–81. Retrieved from https://jarm.journals.yorku.ca/index.php/jarm/article/view/40554

Caldwell, C.M. (2016). Body identity development: Definitions and discussions. *Body, Movement and Dance in Psychotherapy, 11*(4), 220–234. 10.1080/17432979.2016.1145141

Caldwell, C.M. (2018a). *Bodyfulness. Somatic practices for presence, empowerment, and waking up in this life*. Shambala.

Caldwell, C.M. (2018b). Body identity development: Who we are and who we become. In C.M. Caldwell, & L.B. Leighton (Eds.), *Oppression and the body. Roots, resistance, and resolutions* (pp. 31–50). North Atlantic Books.

Caldwell, C.M., & Leighton, L.B. (Eds.). (2018). *Oppression and the body. Roots, resistance, and resolutions*. North Atlantic Books.

Ennis, L.R. (2014). Intensive mothering. Revisiting the issue today. In L.R. Ennis (Ed.), *Intensive mothering: The cultural contradictions of modern motherhood* (pp. 1–23). Demeter Press.

Garland McKinney, J.L., & Meinersmann, L.M. (2022). The cost of intersectionality: Motherhood, mental health, and the state of the country. *Journal of Social Issues, 00*, 1–21. 10.1111/josi.12539

Green, F.J. (2004). Feminist mothers: Successfully negotiating the tensions between motherhood and mothering. In A. O'Reilly (Ed.), *Mother outlaws: Theories and practices of empowered mothering* (pp. 31–42). Women's Press.

Green, F.J. (2009). *Feminist mothering in theory and practice, 1985-1995: A study in transformative politics*. The Edwin Mellen Press.

Green, F.J. (2019). Practicing matricentric feminist mothering. *Journal of the Motherhood Initiative for Research & Community Involvement, 10*(1/2), 83–99. Retrieved from https://jarm.journals.yorku.ca/index.php/jarm/article/view/40555

Hays, S. (1996). *The cultural contradictions of motherhood*. Yale University Press.

Henderson, A., Harmon, S., and Newman, H. (2016). The price mothers pay, even when they are not buying it: Mental health consequences of idealized motherhood. *Sex Roles, 74*, 512–526. 10.1007/s11199-015-0534-5

Laing, O. (2021). *Everybody. A book about freedom*. W.W. Norton.

Leighton, L.B. (2018). The trauma of oppression: A somatic perspective. In C.M. Caldwell, & L.B. Leighton (Eds.), *Oppression and the body. Roots, resistance, and resolutions* (pp. 17–30). North Atlantic Books.

Liss, M., Schiffrin, H.H., & Rizzo, K.M. (2012). Maternal guilt and shame: The role of self-discrepancy and fear of negative evaluation. *Journal of Child and Family Studies, 22*, 1112–1119. 10.1007/s10826-012-9673-2

Little, M.O., & Wickremsinhe, M.N. (2017). Research with pregnant women: A call to action. *Reproductive Health, 14*(3), 156. 10.1186/s12978-017-0419-x

McCarthy, M., Houghton, C., & Matvienko-Sikar, K. (2021). Women's experiences and perceptions of anxiety and stress during the perinatal period: A systematic review and qualitative evidence synthesis. *BMC Pregnancy Childbirth, 21*(1), 811. 10.1186/s12884-021-04271-w

Meeussen, L., & Van Laar, C. (2018). Feeling pressure to be a perfect mother relates to parental burnout and career ambitions. *Frontiers in Psychology, 9*, 2113. 10.3389/fpsyg.2018.02113

O'Brien Hallstein, L. (2015). *Bikini-ready moms. Celebrity profiles, motherhood, and the body*. State University of New York Press.

O'Reilly, A. (2007). Feminist mothering. In A. O'Reilly (Ed.), *Maternal theory. Essential readings* (pp. 792–821). Demeter Press.

O'Reilly, A. (2019). Matricentric feminism: A feminism for mothers. *Journal of the Motherhood Initiative for Research and Community Involvement, 10*(1/2). Retrieved from https://jarm.journals.yorku.ca/index.php/jarm/article/view/40551

O'Reilly, A. (2020). Maternal theory: Patriarchal motherhood and empowered mothering. In L. O'Brien Hallstein, A. O'Reilly, & M.V. Giles (Eds.), *The Routledge companion to motherhood* (pp. 19–35). Routledge. 10.4324/9781315167848

O'Reilly, A. (2021). *Matricentric feminism. Theory, activism, practice. The 2nd edition.* Demeter Press. 10.2307/j.ctv1k2j331

Parker, R. (1995). *Mother love/mother hate. The power of maternal ambivalence.* BasicBooks.

Rich, A. (1976). *Of women born: Motherhood as experience and institution.* W.W.Norton.

Rizzo, K.M., Schiffrin, H.H., & Liss, M. (2012). Insight into the parenthood paradox: Mental health outcomes of intensive mothering. *Journal of Child and Family Studies, 22*, 614–620. 10.1007/s10826-012-9615-z

Ruddick, S. (1989). *Maternal thinking: Towards a politics of peace.* Beacon Press.

Sockol, L.E., Epperson, C.N., & Barber, J.P. (2014). The relationship between maternal attitudes and symptoms of depression and anxiety among pregnant and postpartum first-time mothers. *Archives of Women's Mental Health, 17*(3), 199–212. 10.1007/s00737-014-0424-9

Stone, A. (2014). Psychoanalysis and maternal subjectivity. In P. Bueskens (Ed.), *Mothering and psychoanalysis: Clinical, sociological, and feminist perspectives* (pp. 325–342). Demeter Press.

Vissing, H. (2014). The ideal mother fantasy and its protective function. In L. Ennis (Ed.), *Intensive mothering: The cultural contradictions of modern motherhood* (pp. 104–119). Demeter Press.

Warner, J. (2005). *Perfect madness: Motherhood in the age of anxiety.* Riverhead Books.

4

Rationale and Principles of Somatic Maternal Healing

From Top-Down to Bottom-Up: Neuroscientific Advances in Traumatology

Findings from psychological, biomedical, and social sciences make it clear that we cannot ignore the role of the body in trauma treatment or the maternal transition. The many risk factors at play in Maternal Mental Health interact in complex ways that we do not yet have exhaustive explanations for. However, they do manifest in concrete ways in the body and nervous system through dynamics we have a developed understanding of through affect regulation research, interpersonal neurobiology, and traumatology. Somatic psychology and body-based interventions have developed from these neuroscience advances showing that subcortical brain levels are implicated in trauma reactions making it necessary to apply bottom-up interventions that target the psychophysiological reactions to trauma.

Around the mid-1980s, psychotherapy underwent a shift from subject-object thinking towards understanding the therapeutic relationship as a two-subject interaction, often called "the relational turn" (Beebe & Lachmann, 2003). Given the magnitude and growth of the nervous system and affect regulation research over the last 30 years (Schore, 2012) and how this

DOI: 10.4324/9781003310914-6

research has significantly influenced clinical interventions (see Levine, 2010 and van der Kolk, 2015), it is warranted to recognize that a new shift has been and still is underway, from a top-down mentalization-focused perspective towards a bottom-up perspective that acknowledges the primacy of the body and nervous system in psychotherapy. As mentioned in Chapter 1, the growth of the field of body-focused psychotherapy was made possible in part by the relational turn in psychoanalysis, but also due to the significant advances in the neuroscientific fields of interpersonal neurobiology, affect regulation theory, and traumatology. SAMHSA (2014) has recognized how advances in neuroscience and trauma biology have contributed to the emergence of a biopsychosocial understanding of trauma. The shift towards the bottom-up perspective has forced psychotherapy in general – and trauma treatment in particular – to develop a new understanding of the therapeutic relationship as one of coregulation, in LaPierre's words, "an attuned and collaborative relational matrix" (2015, p. 1). Not only psychoanalysis, but most schools of psychotherapy now acknowledge the role of nonverbal communication in the therapeutic relationship (Schore, 2021). The developments in neuroscience have made it impossible to adopt an affect regulation approach to psychotherapy without acknowledging the intersubjective nature of our nervous systems. Intersubjective relating is now understood as interactions between bodily states of arousal (Hill, 2015).

As it has become widely acknowledged in the scientific literature that affects have a bodily foundation (Levine, 2010; Schore, 2012; van der Kolk, 2015), it follows that we also acknowledge that affect regulation is effective regulation of the body (Hill, 2015). Core therapeutic concepts like empathy, congruence, and attunement are now explored from both the level of mentalization and the level of nervous system regulation. Affect regulation research has demonstrated that regulation is primary and mentalization is secondary (Hill, 2015). Attunement is described by Schore (2012) as "synchronicity of affect states" between individuals and as a growth-promoting psychobiological phenomenon. The coordination of the mother's responsiveness shapes the development of the infant's regulatory capacity, thus making regulation a co-created experience for the mother and infant (Ostlund et al., 2017). The attunement of sharing affect states has a regulating effect even when we share negative affect (Hill, 2015). Beebe et al.'s (2012) comprehensive mother-infant research has demonstrated that it is the caregiver's mirroring of namely distress that is crucial for the infant's self-regulation development; if the caregiver responds to the infant's distress with positive expressiveness or surprise, the infant may experience this as a form of "denial" of their affect. Lack of affect attunement is a hallmark of insecure and disorganized attachment, now broadly understood as synonymous with attachment or developmental trauma. Schore (2021) has also addressed the role of attunement to negative affect in his research; the intersubjective nonverbal communications of interests and feelings between infant and caregiver, including negative affect, allow for the experience of synchronized sharing of affect which is crucial for the development of regulation capacities. The ability of the dyad to share affect states is foundational for activating caregiver responsiveness: Babies express distress because they need to elicit a response from the caregiver. Negative affect must be intersubjectively shared for evolutionary purposes.

Interpersonal neurobiology research shows that intersubjective communication – the constant synchronized nonverbal coregulating exchanges – is not just between minds but between bodies. Schore (2021) emphasizes that the foundation of interpersonal synchrony is the alignment between the bodies of the mother of the infant in "face-to-face protoconversations" (p. 1). These insights have informed the bottom-up approaches that not only include but center nervous system coregulation dynamics in psychotherapy. Bottom-up approaches focus on subcortical brain level processing and the nervous system patterns and body states related to it (Kuhfuß et al., 2021). Body-centered psychotherapy based on the bottom-up approach is therefore characterized by centering the primacy of right-hemispheric processing, the client and therapist's embodiment, and working relationally through attunement to establish congruency between the verbal narrative and the state of the body (Mortimore, 2022). Body-centered psychotherapy is also distinguished by its centering on somatic sensory experiences in all aspects of treatment (Kaplan & Schwartz, 2005). When bodily resonance and affect attunement are applied as central clinical tools to build rapport, the therapeutic effect of empathy becomes more complex and addresses the client's sense of self (LaPierre, 2015). Coregulation and attunement are foundational to subjectivity (Schore, 2021). It is through the regulation of affect states that the sense of self emerges, thus working with attunement in the relational matrix is key when working to "facilitate the emergence of Self" (LaPierre, 2015, p. 1). Because of the neuroscientific insights about the relational and psychobiological nature of subjectivity, the turn towards bottom-up interventions has not only emphasized the importance of the therapeutic relationship but changed our understanding of it: The therapist does not only facilitate new insights for the client through trust, empathic bonding, and analytic interpretations, but is an active participant in the intersubjective coregulating co-construction of the relationship with the client. This requires the therapist to provide nonverbal experiences of relational safety and attunement to the client's affect. Lack of safety impacts our sense of agency and therefore limits our capacities for making changes (Hill, 2015). In somatic interventions, it is the therapist's embodied presence that is the primary tool for creating relational safety (Falls, 2022).

The Bottom-Up Approach to Trauma Treatment: The Scientific Background for Somatic Psychotherapy

Top-down approaches focus on cognitions: How thoughts influence emotions and behaviors. They target distorted beliefs and maladaptive behaviors by creating more adaptive self-beliefs. This intervention relies on insight. The impact of trauma on cognitive functioning may reduce the efficacy of cognitively based treatment for some trauma survivors (Kuhfuß et al., 2021). Bottom-up approaches begin with focusing on the body and nervous system responses to trauma and from there work towards higher cortical functioning (Levine, 2010; van der Kolk, 2015). This is based on the principle that instinctual shock states must be addressed before cognition or affect can be effectively worked with as a traumatized brain flooded by lower brain activation is not able to access cognition effectively (Levine et al., 2018; van der Kolk, 2015). The main issue of PTSD is dysregulation of arousal modulation (Schore, 2012; van der Kolk, 2015). The neurological structures of dysregulation involve the so-called "lower" parts of the brain, the corticolimbic system. Interventions that target body and physical sensations and nonverbal affect regulation first are therefore appropriate for treating issues of arousal and regulation (Levine, 2010; van der Kolk, 2015). The bottom-up approach addresses the sensory level of symptoms first.

One of the primary schools of bottom-up trauma treatment, Somatic Experiencing® (SE), was developed by Levine (1997, 2010) who was inspired by his studies of wild animals and their responses to stressors. Levine's (2010) model of SE emphasizes that the advances in neuroscience and human biology research on trauma have revealed that the psychobiological systems involved in trauma responses are also the foundation of our general sense of goodness, vitality, and connectedness. In SE, trauma symptoms are treated by changing interoceptive and proprioceptive sensations associated with the traumatic experience so that freeze responses are uncoupled from overwhelming fear and subsequently processed by completion of the nervous system activation cycle (Kuhfuß et al., 2021; Levine, 2010; Payne et al., 2015). The primary point of intervention is therefore sensations, the client's awareness of and relationship with sensations, i.e., regulation. The primary goal of SE is to modify the stress response to the trauma by firstly helping the client increase tolerance for the arousal associated with the trauma with internal and external resources of sensory awareness, and secondly to guide the client carefully through a discharge process that facilitates completion and renegotiation of the nervous system survival response (Levine, 2010; Payne et al., 2015). The physiological trauma impulses are resolved by integrating them into the therapeutic process. As a bottom-up approach, SE is focused on the client's self-regulation capacities and can therefore be used to treat other conditions of dysregulation that are not directly trauma-related (Kuhfuß et al., 2021). Bottom-up approaches can also be used in conjunction with or as an addition to other cognitive-behavioral modalities (van de Kamp, 2019). It is important to note that SE is not a form of exposure therapy as it specifically avoids direct and overwhelming re-telling of traumatic events (Payne et al., 2015). From the bottom-up approach, SE is focused on the gradual integration of traumatic memories through titrated processing of dysregulation and survival responses (Levine, 2010; Levine et al., 2018).

Schore's (2013) comprehensive research on the interpersonal neurobiological model of intersubjectivity demonstrates how nervous system dysregulation is at the core of trauma psychopathology. A central principle of bottom-up clinical interventions for trauma is that the clinician continuously works towards shifting from explicit left brain relating (verbal analytic) to implicit right brain interactions through attunement, to facilitate the client's regulation in a co-created way (Hill, 2015; Schore, 2021). Concretely this means that bottom-up approaches continuously prioritize nonverbal attunement and coregulation, as the basis for any subsequent processing of affect or cognition. The therapeutic relationship becomes effective only when safety is established through coregulation (Geller & Porges, 2014; Porges, 2022). Through therapeutic presence, the therapist communicates safety by expressing nonverbal signals of social engagement and thereby down-regulates the nervous systems of both therapist and client. The autonomic nervous system functions from ongoing safety appraisal that determines whether it is safe for the person to engage socially (Porges, 2022). Therapeutic coregulation is therefore contingent upon the therapist's ability to establish and communicate safety from an authentically regulated state. Cues of coregulation of autonomic nervous system functioning are offered through voice, gesture, and facial expression (Jokić et al., 2022). The starting point of somatic psychology is the therapist's self-regulation capacities. A recent study by Jokić et al. (2022) demonstrated that body psychotherapists had better autonomic nervous system functioning than the general population despite having higher rates of childhood maltreatment, indicating the positive benefits of somatic training focusing on autonomic nervous system functioning.

Despite increasing clinical use, bottom-up approaches to psychotherapy that focus on the body are neglected in scientific literature and research (Rosendahl et al., 2021). The evidence base for body-focused bottom-up psychotherapy is challenged by an imbalance between a significant amount of evidence for the underlying principles and few efficacy and effectiveness studies. As reviewed above, there is significant evidence for the principles of bottom-up somatic approaches, especially from the field of interpersonal neurobiology (Schore, 2021), but only emerging evidence on the efficacy using the golden standard of Randomized Controlled Trials (RCTs). In their systematic review and meta-analysis, van de Kamp et al. (2019) demonstrated that combining Body- and Movement-Oriented Interventions (BMOIs) with other psychotherapy treatments or using BMOIs alone may be effective in reducing PTSD symptoms and comorbid depression. This study examined a broad range of BMOIs and did not produce evidence for specific somatic techniques. However, the results support the hypothesis that given the neurological impact of trauma, bottom-up interventions that target affect regulation are important for PTSD treatment. In a recent systematic review and meta-analysis of RCT studies of a wide range of body-focused psychotherapies, Rosendahl et al. (2021) also demonstrated a medium effect size on primary outcomes of psychopathology and psychological distress, indicating non-neglectable evidence for effectiveness. Although limited, some RCT studies of SE exist. The first RCT study on efficacy (Brom et al., 2017) demonstrated a large effect size on PTSD and depression symptoms, indicating that SE is likely an effective treatment for PTSD. A limitation of RCT studies on SE lies in the organic nature of the modality where the clinician addresses the client's symptoms of dysregulation directly as they manifest experientially in session, as opposed to manualized or protocol-based interventions (Brom et al., 2017).

There is an acute need for high-quality efficacy and effectiveness studies in the entire field of body psychotherapy

(Rosendahl et al., 2021). The specific factors and mechanisms of the therapeutic alliance in somatic modalities have not been studied with the RCT standard yet. A consistent and widely acknowledged finding from decades of psychotherapy research is that the therapeutic alliance is the most important predictor of positive outcomes of psychotherapy (Norcross & Lambert, 2019). The therapeutic presence that emerges from the therapist's intentional use of coregulation and attunement to connect with the client has been explained from the neuroscientific well-researched framework of polyvagal theory (Geller & Porges, 2014). This analysis indicates that the neurological states of experiencing safety are central to the relational safety that is necessary for a therapeutic alliance. Somatic approaches focus on establishing and cultivating the embodied experience of relational safety. The comprehensive training in autonomic nervous system regulation that somatic therapists go through enables them to apply interventions of coregulation of the neural social engagement systems of the client and therapist (Jokić et al., 2022).

It is important to note that while several modalities for the treatment of PTSD and other forms of trauma have been studied thoroughly and their effectiveness has been demonstrated, no single method has been demonstrated to work for all people suffering from PTSD (Brom et al., 2017; Granner & Seng, 2021). This points to the wide variations of how trauma manifests depending on the population and contexts and the subsequent need for specialized modalities that are formed around the unique needs of the client population. As seen in the literature, somatic bottom-up approaches are highly relevant to the treatment of trauma. However, when we review the particular conditions of the perinatal period, the unique psychobiological changes of the maternal transition, and its complex connection to trauma, the need for a somatic approach becomes even more evident.

The Heightened Risks for Trauma in the Perinatal Period

As discussed in Chapter 2, pregnancy and the postpartum period impact several biological systems that are highly sensitive to stress and trauma, including inflammatory responses, hormonal systems like oxytocin and cortisol, the HPA axis, and catecholamine responses. These systems are highly sensitive to stress, both directly during the perinatal period, and indirectly through the impacts of a mother's early life adversity and developmental trauma. While the research on biomarkers for PMADs is promising, there are no specific biomarker screenings ready for clinical use (Guintivano et al., 2018). The current best predictors of PMADs are psychiatric history and history of adverse life events (Guintivano et al., 2018), emphasizing the centrality of trauma and accumulated allostatic load as risk factors. The perinatal period is also characterized by a significant increase in several forms of stress like lack of sleep, less time for self-care, and intensification of social attunement work. The combined increase in stressors likely makes it harder for mothers to maintain usual coping strategies that otherwise work as trauma buffers (Choi & Sikkema, 2016). The usual resilience that can prevent or lessen the overwhelm and stress associated with trauma might be lowered by perinatal stress, especially in combination with a lack of social support. The biological impact of previous trauma also puts the expecting or new mother at risk for new trauma due to long-term or chronic medical consequences (allostatic load), including complex medical conditions like autoimmune diseases and chronic pain. The perinatal period is a time of considerable strain on not only psychological and social levels, but of a woman's entire biology and its complex interactions with her mental and emotional health.

The general prevalence of anxiety is higher in the perinatal period compared to other times in women's lives (Pawluski et al., 2017). A mother's concerns about her baby's vulnerability are not only normal but also adaptive elements of the maternal transition, but at high levels, they can contribute to maladaptive anxiety (Pawluski et al., 2017). This could put the expecting or new mother at higher risk for trauma given that pre-trauma anxiety is associated with PTSD reactions (Sareen, 2014). Heightened anxiety, even when adaptive, increases the risk for newly isolated trauma as well as re-activation of previous trauma. As mentioned in Chapter 2, the increase in oxytocin following birth enables mothers to be highly attuned to social cues, but also creates a challenge of increased sensitivity to misattunements from the surroundings (Kendall-Tackett, 2019), which can activate attachment trauma reactivity. The maternal transition requires robust self-regulation to handle the increase in anxiety.

Attachment and relational functioning undergo major reorganizing during the transition to motherhood which creates heightened vulnerability to the reactivation of emotions and memories related to childhood adverse experiences. This reorganization creates a vulnerability for new relational trauma, stress, or activation of childhood maltreatment. Namely childhood maltreatment, which impacts attachment development, is recognized as a strong predictor of pregnancy PTSD (Cook et al., 2018), with cumulative sociodemographic factors exacerbating risk (Seng et al., 2009). The increased dependency on support for practical and emotional reasons makes the new mother vulnerable to the stress of lack of support, evidence by the consistent research findings that social support is a significant protective factor against PMADs (Feinberg et al., 2022) and that symptoms of PMADs are inversely associated with social support (Milgrom et al., 2019). The perinatal period requires extra social and community support, which is often lacking, especially for vulnerable groups and parents from minority backgrounds. The lack of support on community and systemic levels during a time with higher needs for support increases the vulnerability of the perinatal period.

It is also important to consider the iatrogenic components of trauma in the perinatal period as it is a time with a high frequency of invasive medical interventions. Pregnancy, delivery, and postpartum involve extensive medical interventions and therefore also risks of iatrogenic trauma or "intervention cascades" that put the mother at risk for trauma both medically speaking and from a mental health perspective. Because of the intensity of medical interventions, mothers with a trauma history are at heightened risk for re-traumatization or re-activation of previous trauma (Seng & Taylor, 2015), particularly sexual abuse survivors (Beck et al. 2013; Simkin & Klaus, 2004) and childhood maltreatment survivors (Choi & Sikkema, 2016). Autonomic nervous system functioning will influence a woman's reactions to the comprehensive and invasive medical interventions of the perinatal period. Whether a woman has pre-existing trauma or accumulated stress, or she is experiencing new trauma or traumatic stress during her maternal transition, her autonomic nervous system functioning is a central factor in her coping.

As discussed in Chapter 3, any aspect of the perinatal transition, including trauma biology related to obstetric interventions, cannot be understood outside of systemic and social contexts of health inequity and discrimination. We have an abundance of deeply concerning data demonstrating disparities in perinatal care. Particularly women of color experience healthcare inequities (Bryant et al., 2010), have higher risks for adverse birth outcomes including infant and maternal mortality (Douthard et al., 2021) and preterm birth (Culhane & Goldenberg, 2011), and have a higher prevalence of PMADs and PTSD (Orr et al., 2006; Kornfield et al., 2022). It is crucial that clinicians avoid pathologizing the individual by applying isolated trauma biology analysis of the individual mother who is subjected to systemic discrimination and poor quality of medical care. Rage, anger, mistrust, and hypervigilance can be understood as trauma reactions (Levine, 2010), but biopsychosocial and trauma-informed clinical thinking that takes societal contexts into consideration will also understand such reactions as normal responses to social injustices, health inequity, and actual threats against one's safety. The concept of betrayal trauma has been developed to include institutional betrayal, which is the wrongdoings by institutions that individuals depend on (Smith & Freyd, 2014). Betrayal trauma is characterized by a violation of trust. It is this violation of trust in a necessary relationship that makes betrayal trauma particularly harmful (Freyd, 1996). The disparities in Maternal Mental Health reflect a form of institutional betrayal. From a matricentric feminist perspective, this betrayal can be understood as a result of patriarchal motherhood dynamics.

Because of these complex interacting factors, the perinatal period is a time of increased vulnerability to trauma and thus an increased need for trauma-informed bottom-up interventions that focus on coregulation and nervous system support. Perinatal trauma causes significant rippling consequences for the mother, the child, the family, the community, and ultimately society. The permutations of perinatal trauma conditions are sometimes recognized as trauma, sometimes as PMADs, and sometimes seen as "normal" psychosocial stress of parenting. A nervous system-informed approach reframes our understanding of perinatal trauma reactions.

From Vulnerability to Opportunity

Biopsychosocial clinical thinking promotes a shift away from a pathology framework towards an appreciation of the adaptive nature of the perinatal period and thus the potential for healing. The biology of the maternal transition is a time of vulnerability, but also a unique opportunity for preventing, mitigating, circumventing, and transforming the impacts of trauma and traumatic stress patterns (Seng & Taylor, 2015). This is furthered by the philosophy of somatic psychology that recognizes the connection between nervous system regulation trauma treatment with general vitality, self-regulation, and relational capacities (Levine, 2010). The reviewed research points to two intertwined principles for trauma-responsive perinatal interventions: 1) the need to balance the view of the perinatal period as one of the unique vulnerabilities with the appreciation of the unique opportunities for healing because of the plasticity of the maternal brain and nervous system and the coregulatory nature of the perinatal period, and 2) the importance of seizing all opportunities for anti-inflammatory interventions, through both biomedical means and behavioral techniques, especially nervous system regulation. In this context, anti-inflammatory intervention is understood in the broadest way, meaning it includes both acute issues of pain management and treatment of local infections, and general stress-reduction in medical, psychological, and social areas of life as well as disruption of underlying nervous system dysregulation that fuels stress patterns. With this holistic lens, our understanding of trauma is widened. When we recognize the connections between trauma, toxic stress, nervous system dysregulation, lack of relational safety, and inflammation, we expand the clinical perspective from a narrow focus on the PTSD diagnosis or specific acute trauma to a wider perspective of trauma as a continuum of the cumulative burden of chronic stress and life events, also called allostatic load and overload (Guidi et al., 2021). As mentioned, it is a challenge for clinicians to discern normal adjustment reactions to the intensity of the maternal transition from trauma reactions. However, a mother's coregulatory functioning is a helpful proxy for her accumulated trauma and stress impact (including allostatic load and overload) as it is a central factor in her parenting, her experience of any trauma and mental health disorders, and the prognosis for treatment.

This widened understanding of trauma has implications for clinical language and treatment strategies. The term "trauma" is not always adequate or appropriate when working with the many layers of perinatal trauma. Allostatic load is a clinical and technical term that is helpful for treatment conceptualization and research, but it may not be appropriate to use with some clients. Other terms to consider are overwhelm, dysregulation, upheaval, adjustment stress, traumatic stress, or stress imprints. The advantage of a trauma-informed approach that broadens the understanding of trauma is that "too much" trauma-informed care does not present risks of harm to clients with very little allostatic load or who do not have a trauma history, if the language used with clients is appropriately adapted. Those clients can still benefit from the principles of trauma-informed care, and the principles still serve the crucial function of prevention of new-onset trauma which is of acute concern for the perinatal population (Polmanteer et al., 2019; Seng & Taylor, 2015). Autonomic nervous system regulation is also beneficial for people who do not have a severe trauma history.

The Rationale for Somatic Interventions in Maternal Mental Health

Despite the high prevalence of trauma in the perinatal period and the acute concerns about the links between PTSD during pregnancy and adverse birth outcomes, studies on the treatment of PTSD during pregnancy are scarce (Stevens et al., 2020). In their systematic review of studies focusing on the treatment of perinatal anxiety and trauma-related disorders, Nillni et al. (2018) identified a tremendous need for more research in this area. Most studies on the treatment of PMADs focus on the treatment of Postpartum Depression and there is thus a gap in knowledge on the treatment of perinatal anxiety and trauma-related disorders (Nillni et al., 2018). It is therefore timely to develop a somatic approach to Maternal Mental Health. It is well-established that trauma and traumatic stressors are significant risk factors for PMADs (Grekin et al., 2017; Seng & Taylor, 2015). Generally, for trauma treatment, the importance of bottom-up approaches is also widely recognized (Schore, 2012, 2021). Several points form the rationale basis for somatic interventions for perinatal trauma treatment including the prevalence of perinatal trauma, the heightened vulnerability to the impact of trauma in the perinatal period reviewed above, the coregulatory nature of mothering. Coregulation-focused interventions like somatic psychotherapy integrated with psychodynamic psychotherapy also have the advantage of engaging the potential for deeper trauma healing imbedded in the maternal transition: The revisiting of relational dynamics and reworking of subjectivity and an embodied sense of self in the process of maternal identity development. This offers an opportunity to work through components of developmental trauma related to the sense of self not only on a cognitive level but also on an intersubjective affect regulation level.

The need for interventions aimed at treating trauma-related disorders of the perinatal period combined with the reviewed risks, opportunities, and unique characteristics of the maternal transition all point to the potential for bottom-up somatic interventions in trauma-responsive Maternal Mental Health. Although all therapeutic work must include a balance of mentalization-based insight and affect attunement, perinatal work requires a heavy emphasis on the primacy of coregulation because the postpartum phase is 1) a time of high trauma-vulnerability and 2) a realm of constant nonverbal coregulation work of attunement and forming attachments with a baby. My aim here is not to use the infant's development as the main argument for somatic coregulation-focused interventions with mothers, as this would be a reiteration of the child-centric attitude that perpetuates the othering and erasure of maternal subjectivity discussed in Chapter 1 and the oppressive dynamics of patriarchal motherhood that produce maternal bodylessness discussed in Chapter 3. Somatic interventions in Maternal Mental Health address the coregulation needs and experiences of the new mother who is doing the intense work of constant nonverbal attunement, especially in the context of trauma, which is an acute concern in the perinatal period.

Somatic psychology aims to build a client's regulation capacities as a central part of the resolution of trauma. Mothering is inherently demanding on emotional and physical levels: It is indeed the way emotional and physical self-regulation are intertwined and intensified in the caretaking of an infant that makes mothering demanding, even more so with a trauma history. Interventions that do not acknowledge and address the coregulation aspects of the postpartum period will at best not help the mother reduce her anxiety and other symptoms that are impacting her coregulation and nervous system functioning, and at worst can exacerbate her coregulation issues, especially if the therapeutic relationship is causing unaddressed misattunements and ruptures that contribute to her distress. For some mothers, ruptures by a therapist can contribute to trauma reactions, especially mothers with relationship trauma. Trauma-focused interventions that have a narrow focus on only resolving specific traumatic memories miss out on the opportunities for supporting the new mother's general regulation capacities, which are crucial in her maternal transition. The focus on self-regulation in somatic psychology is important for asserting embodied maternal subjectivity (discussed in Chapter 1) and addressing issues of maternal bodylessness (discussed in Chapter 3).

The biopsychosocial adaptations of the perinatal period make it a time of heightened vulnerable to trauma, but it also offers a unique opportunity for deeper trauma healing work –

this potential can only be fully unlocked if the body and nervous system are brought into the treatment. The stress of the coregulation work of mothering is not only to be endured but can become central to the healing of the dysregulation patterns of trauma, in the context of an attuned and coregulating therapeutic relationship. Furthermore, when applied with ordinary standards of care and clinical trauma-sensitivity that prevent and reduce overwhelm and focus on the client's resources for self-regulation, somatic interventions are not inherently invasive or aggressive in nature and therefore do not pose significant risks of harm. Somatic modalities are inherently formed towards preventing overwhelm for the client with sensory awareness tracking skills (addressed in Chapter 5). Somatic psychotherapy is not automatically an exposure technique and does not require detailed narrating of the traumatic events that may cause overwhelm. On the contrary, a somatic approach emphasizes slowing down the pace of the client's activation by monitoring arousal and downregulating it, thereby preventing excessive overwhelm (Brom et al., 2017; Levine, 2010). This approach is useful for the perinatal period, which is characterized by high levels of stress and significant barriers to treatment.

Integrating Psychodynamic Psychotherapy and Somatic Psychotherapy

As the examination of feminist psychoanalytic literature in Chapter 1 demonstrated, the experience of the maternal transition is a position that is inherently challenging to articulate and acknowledge due to the elusiveness of maternal subjectivity and its radical transformation of embodiment. Much is lost in translation when we attempt to articulate the maternal experience. The maternal transition is an experience primarily of the bodily realm; the realm of nonverbal viscerality and corporeal sensory profundity. Trauma can cause a destabilization of the sense of self. The maternal transition also carries a destabilization of the sense of self, in intertwined psychological and somatic ways where the body-self undergoes dramatic upheaval. The mother who carries a trauma history or who experiences trauma in her maternal transition (or both) is twice exposed. She is therefore in particular need of care and treatment that addresses the magnitude of this convergence of somatic pressures and acknowledges the nonverbal aspects of the maternal transition. A combined psychodynamic and somatic approach does this by supporting the mother in discovering and integrating her new maternal subjectivity in an embodied relational way, beyond the limitations of verbal work, while treating trauma from a bottom-up approach. Somatic listening skills of attunement and coregulation are also ways of "listening with the body", expanding the range of what can be communicated between therapist and client. When we listen with the body, we are more likely to listen to what is not being said out loud. In this way, the somatic approach is inherently conducive to the psychoanalytic mode of "listening with the third ear".

Relational psychoanalysis and relational body psychotherapy can mutually enrich each other (LaPierre, 2015). Levine, the creator of SE, celebrates the integration of his approach into all healing traditions, including psychodynamic psychotherapy, and has expressed support for the clinical application between the complementary practices of SE and psychoanalysis (Levine et al., 2018). The integrated somatic and psychodynamic approach is useful in that the limitations of language do not hinder the work. Simultaneously, the language used in therapy is expanded by the appreciation of the meaningfulness of sensations and bodily experiences. Working with the complex interplay between the experiential and somatic levels and the narrative verbal levels allows for integration and processing of the subjective experience of the maternal transition, including recent and previous trauma experiences and unconscious material. The somatic approach is helpful because it engages the language of the body, which is sensations (Caldwell, 2018), while acknowledging the interplay between verbal and nonverbal levels of processing. Developing vocabulary related to sensory awareness promotes regulation (Caldwell, 2018; Levine, 2010) while also stimulating the integration of unconscious material. Working with trauma in the maternal transition requires sensitivity to the unique verbal and nonverbal aspects of perinatal sensory awareness (addressed in Chapter 6).

Psychodynamic psychotherapy that minimizes or does not recognize the body has a risk of reducing all symptoms to purely metaphorical phenomena, which is problematic because of the relational nature of the body and all bodily experiences (Orbach, 2006). Integrating a focus on the body indeed furthers the psychodynamic goal of illuminating and integrating the unconscious through a relational process: The complementary perspectives of client and therapist on the client's body as subject and object respectively stimulate the revelation of the unconscious in an intersubjective way (Rosendahl et al., 2021). The integration of the somatic approach with psychodynamic psychotherapy is founded on their shared emphasis on bottom-up processing of affect and the intersubjective nature of bodily experiences. The focus on the bodily experience that somatic psychology offers addresses the central issue of recognition of maternal embodied subjectivity that feminist psychoanalysis reveals.

References

Beebe, B., & Lachmann, F. (2003). The relational turn in psychoanalysis. A dyadic systems view from infant research. *Contemporary Psychoanalysis, 39*(3), 379–409. 10.1080/00107530.2003.10747213

Beebe, B., Lachmann, F., Markese, S., Buck, K.A., Bahrick, L.E., Chen, H., Cohen, P., Andrews, H., Feldstein, S., & Jaffe, J. (2012). On the origins of disorganized attachment and internal working models: Paper II. An empirical microanalysis of 4-month mother-infant interaction. *Psychoanalytic Dialogues, 22*(3), 352–374. 10.1080/10481885.2012.679606

Beck, C.T., Driscoll, J.W., & Watson, S. (2013). *Traumatic childbirth* (1st ed.). Routledge. 10.4324/9780203766699

Brom, D., Stokar, Y., Lawi, C., Nuriel-Porat, V., Ziv, Y., Lerner, K., & Ross, G. (2017). Somatic experiencing for posttraumatic stress disorder: A randomized controlled outcome study. *Journal of Traumatic Stress, 0,* 1–9. 10.1002/jts.22189

Bryant, A.S., Worjoloh, A., Caughey, A.B., & Washington, A.E. (2010). Racial/ethnic disparities in obstetric outcomes and care: Prevalence and determinants. *American Journal of Obstetrics and Gynecology, 202*(4), 335–343. 10.1016/j.ajog.2009.10.864

Caldwell, C.M. (2018). *Bodyfulness. Somatic practices for presence, empowerment, and waking up in this life.* Shambala.

Choi, K.W., & Sikkema, K.J. (2016). Childhood maltreatment and perinatal mood and anxiety disorders: A systematic review. *Trauma, Violence & Abuse, 17*(5), 427–453. 10.1177/1524838015584369

Cook, N., Ayers, S., & Horsch, A. (2018). Maternal posttraumatic stress disorder during the perinatal period and child outcomes: A systematic review. *Journal of Affective Disorders, 225,* 18–31. 10.1016/j.jad.2017.07.045

Culhane, J.F., & Goldenberg, R.L. (2011). Racial disparities in preterm birth. *Seminars in Perinatology, 35*(4), 234–239. 10.1053/j.semperi.2011.02.020

Douthard, R.A., Martin, I.K., Chapple-McGruder, T., Langer, A., & Chang, S. (2021). U.S. maternal mortality within a global context: Historical trends, current state, and future directions. *Journal of Women's Health (2002), 30*(2), 168–177. 10.1089/jwh.2020.8863

Falls, N. (2022). Embodied presence. The essential therapeutic stance in working with addictive behaviors. *International Body Psychotherapy Journal, 21*(1), 32–42.

Feinberg, E., Declercq, E., Lee, A., & Belanoff, C. (2022). The relationship between social support and postnatal anxiety and depression: Results from the listening to mothers in California survey. *Women's Health issues: Official publication of the Jacobs Institute of Women's Health, 32*(3), 251–260. 10.1016/j.whi.2022.01.005

Freyd, J.J. (1996). *Betrayal trauma: The logic of forgetting childhood abuse.* Harvard University Press.

Geller, S.M., & Porges, S.W. (2014). Therapeutic presence: Neurophysiological mechanisms mediating feeling safe in therapeutic relationships. *Journal of Psychotherapy Integration, 24*(3), 178–192. 10.1037/a0037511

Granner, J.R., & Seng, J.S. (2021). Using theories of posttraumatic stress to inform perinatal care clinician responses to trauma reactions.

Journal of Midwifery & Women's Health, 66(5), 567–578. 10.1111/jmwh.13287

Grekin, R., Brock, R.L., & O'Hara, M.W. (2017). The effects of trauma on perinatal depression: Examining trajectories of depression from pregnancy through 24 months postpartum in an at-risk population. *Journal of Affective Disorders, 218*, 269–276. 10.1016/j.jad.2017.04.051

Guidi, J., Lucente, M., Sonino, N., & Fava, G.A. (2021). Allostatic load and its impact on health: A systematic review. *Psychotherapy and Psychosomatics, 90*(1), 11–27. 10.1159/000510696

Guintivano, J., Manuck, T., & Meltzer-Brody, S. (2018). Predictors of Postpartum Depression: A comprehensive review of the last decade of evidence. *Clinical Obstetrics and Gynecology, 61*(3), 591–603. 10.1097/GRF.0000000000000368

Hill, D. (2015). *Affect regulation theory. A clinical model.* Norton.

Jokić, B., Purić, D., Grassmann, H., Walling, C.G., Nix, E.J., Porges, S.W., & Kolacz, J. (2022). Association of childhood maltreatment with adult body awareness and autonomic reactivity: The moderating effect of practicing body psychotherapy. *Psychotherapy (Chicago, Ill.)*, 10.1037/pst0000463. Advance online publication. 10.1037/pst0000463

Kaplan, A.H., & Schwartz, L.F. (2005). Listening to the body. Pragmatic case studies of body-centered psychotherapy. *The USA Body Psychotherapy Journal, 4*(2), 23–42.

Kendall-Tackett, K.A. (2019). Creating an oxytocic environment for new mothers. Editorial. *Clinical Lactation, 10*(1), 7–8. 10.1891/2158-0782.10.1.7

Kornfield, S.L., Johnson, R.L., Hantsoo, L.V., Kaminsky, R.B., Waller, R., Sammel, M., & Epperson, C.N. (2022). Engagement in and benefits of a short-term, brief psychotherapy intervention for PTSD during pregnancy. *Frontiers in Psychiatry, 13*, 882429. 10.3389/fpsyt.2022.882429

Kuhfuß, M., Maldei, T., Hetmanek, A., & Baumann, N. (2021). Somatic experiencing – effectiveness and key factors of a body-oriented trauma therapy: A scoping literature review. *European Journal of Psychotraumatology, 12*, 1929023. 10.1080/20008198.2021.1929023

LaPierre, A. (2015). Relational body psychotherapy (or relational somatic psychology). *International Body Psychotherapy Journal*, *14*(2), 80–100.

Levine, P.A. (1997). *Waking the tiger: Healing trauma: The innate capacity to transform overwhelming experiences.* North Atlantic Books.

Levine, P.A. (2010). *In an unspoken voice. How the body releases trauma and restores goodness.* North Atlantic Books.

Levine, P.A., Blakeslee, A., & Sylvae, J. (2018). Reintegrating fragmentation of the primitive self: Discussion of "Somatic Experiencing". *Psychoanalytic Dialogues*, *28*(5), 620–628. 10.1080/10481885.2018.1506216

Milgrom, J., Hirshler, Y., Reece, J., Holt, C., & Gemmill, A.W. (2019). Social support – A protective factor for depressed perinatal women? *International Journal of Environmental Research and Public Health*, *16*(8), 1426. 10.3390/ijerph16081426

Mortimore, L. (2022). Body as portal – bringing the body into practice. *International Body Psychotherapy Journal*, *20*(2), 57–69.

Nillni, Y.I., Mehralizade, A., Mayer, L., & Milanovic, S. (2018). Treatment of depression, anxiety, and trauma-related disorders during the perinatal period: A systematic review. *Clinical Psychology Review*, *66*, 136–148. 10.1016/j.cpr.2018.06.004

Norcross, J.C., & Lambert, M.J. (Eds.). (2019). *Psychotherapy relationships that work: Volume 1: Evidence-based therapist contributions.* Oxford University Press.

Orbach, S. (2006). How can we have a body?: Desires and corporeality. *Studies In Gender & Sexuality*, *7*(1), 89–111.

Orr, S.T., Blazer, D.G., & James, S.A. (2006). Racial disparities in elevated prenatal depressive symptoms among black and white women in eastern North Carolina. *Annals of Epidemiology*, *16*(6), 463–468. 10.1016/j.annepidem.2005.08.004

Ostlund, B.D., Measelle, J.R., Laurent, H.K., Conradt, E., & Ablow, J.C. (2017). Shaping emotion regulation: Attunement, symptomatology, and stress recovery within mother-infant dyads. *Developmental Psychobiology*, *59*(1), 15–25. 10.1002/dev.21448

Pawluski, J.L., Lonstein, J.S., & Fleming, A.S. (2017). The neurobiology of postpartum anxiety and depression. *Trends in Neurosciences*, *40*(2), 106–120. 10.1016/j.tins.2016.11.009

Payne, P., Levine, P.A., & Crane-Godreau, M.A. (2015). Somatic experiencing: Using interoception and proprioception as core elements of trauma therapy. *Frontiers in Psychology, 6*, 93. 10.3389/fpsyg.2015.00093

Polmanteer, R.S.R., Keefe, R.H., & Brownstein-Evans, C. (2019). Trauma-informed care with women diagnosed with postpartum depression: A conceptual framework. *Social Work in Health Care, 58*(2), 220–235. 10.1080/00981389.2018.1535464

Porges, S.W. (2022). Polyvagal theory: A science of safety. *Frontiers in Integrative Neuroscience, 16*, 871227. 10.3389/fnint.2022.871227

Rosendahl, S., Sattel, H., & Lahmann, C. (2021). Effectiveness of body psychotherapy. A systematic review and meta-analysis. *Frontiers in Psychiatry, 12*, 709798. 1–15. 10.3389/fpsyt.2021.709798

Sareen, J. (2014). Posttraumatic stress disorder in adults: Impact, comorbidity, risk factors, and treatment. *The Canadian Journal of Psychiatry, 59*(9), 460–467. 10.1177/070674371405900902

Schore, A.N. (2012). *The science of the art of psychotherapy*. W.W. Norton.

Schore, A.N. (2013). Relational trauma, brain development, and dissociation. In J.D. Ford, & C.A. Courtois (Eds.), *Treating traumatic stress disorders in children and adolescents. Scientific foundations and therapeutic models* (pp. 3–23). Guilford Press.

Schore, A.N. (2021). The interpersonal neurobiology of intersubjectivity. *Frontiers in Psychology, 12*, 648616. 10.3389/fpsyg.2021.648616

Seng, J., & Taylor, J. (Eds.). (2015). *Trauma informed care and the perinatal period*. Dunedin Academic Press.

Seng, J.S., Low, L.K., Sperlich, M., Ronis, D.L., & Liberzon, I. (2009). Prevalence, trauma history, and risk for posttraumatic stress disorder among nulliparous women in maternity care. *Obstetrics and Gynecology, 114*(4), 839–847. 10.1097/AOG.0b013e3181b8f8a2

Simkin, P., & Klaus, P. (2004). *When survivors give birth: Understanding and healing the effects of early sexual abuse on childbearing women*. Classic Day Publishing.

Smith, C.P., & Freyd, J.J. (2014). Institutional betrayal. *American Psychologist, 69*, 575–587. 10.1037/a0037564

Stevens, N.R., Miller, M.L., Soibatian, C., Otwell, C., Rufa, A.K., Meyer, D.J., & Shalowitz, M.U. (2020). Exposure therapy for PTSD during pregnancy: A feasibility, acceptability, and case series study of

Narrative Exposure Therapy (NET). *BMC psychology*, *8*(1), 130. 10.1186/s40359-020-00503-4

Substance Abuse and Mental Health Services Administration. (2014). *SAMHSA's concept of trauma and guidance for a trauma-informed approach*. HHS Publication.

van de Kamp, M.M., Scheffers, M., Hatzmann, J., Emck, C., Cuijpers, P., & Beek, P.J. (2019). Body- and movement-oriented interventions for posttraumatic stress disorder: A systematic review and meta-analysis. *Journal of Traumatic Stress*, *32*(6), 967–976. 10.1002/jts.22465

van der Kolk, B. (2015). *The body keeps the score: Brain, mind, and body in the healing of trauma*. Penguin Publishing.

Introduction to Part II
Principles, Treatment Goals, and Key Clinical Skills of Maternal Somatic Healing

Integrating Feminist Psychoanalysis, Matricentric Feminism, and Somatic Psychology

The importance of claiming and asserting an embodied and coherent sense of self is crucial in the maternal transition, for psychological, social, and somatic reasons. Integrating bodily focused somatic techniques expands the work on maternal identity from mentalization-based second-order changes to bottom-up first-order changes. The nervous system regulation techniques of sensory tracking that are foundational to the somatic treatment of trauma (Levine, 2010) and Caldwell's (2016, 2018a, 2018b) concepts of body identity and bodyfulness do not include analysis of or clinical tools aimed at the specific embodied experience of the maternal transition. It is, therefore, necessary to integrate feminist psychoanalytic thinking to ensure sensitivity to female and maternal embodied subjectivity and a focus on the particular *somatic* manifestations of countertransference when working in the perinatal transferential field.

The matricentric feminist perspective (O'Reilly, 2021) contributes a sociological level of analysis that centers on empowered mothering as a way of resisting patriarchal motherhood through empowered or feminist mothering. It also connects individual trauma treatment to a societal level of activism. Caldwell's (2018b) work also connects the somatic approach with a social perspective in her analysis of how systemic oppressive dynamics impact embodiment and body identity formation.

Somatic Psychology	• Nervous system regulation
Feminist Psychoanalysis	• Assertion of maternal subjectivity • Somatic countertransference
Matricentric Feminism	• Empowered mothering

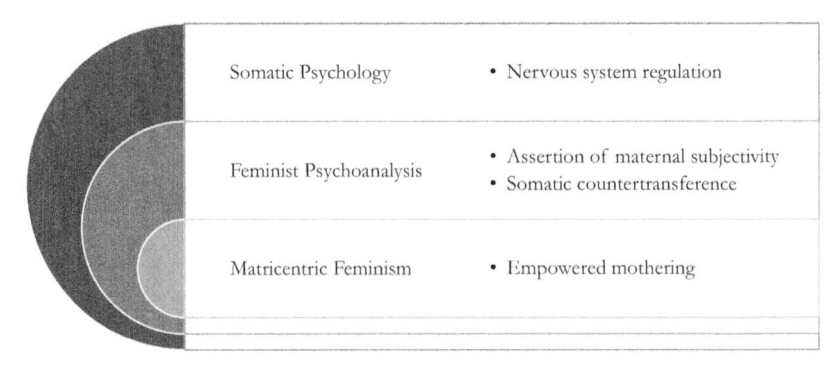

FIGURE 4.1 Integrative Model of Somatic Maternal Healing

The Principles of Somatic Maternal Healing

Somatic Maternal Healing is a framework of biopsychosocially oriented clinical practice (term by Borrell-Carrió et al., 2004) that integrates theory and research from feminist psychoanalysis, somatic psychology, and matricentric feminism (Figure 4.1). The hallmark of this approach is the emphasis on how the different levels interact and overlap, especially in relation to trauma, traumatic stress, and vulnerabilities from the life-long allostatic load. It is therefore important that the following principles based on the theory and research reviewed in Chapters 1–4 are not compartmented or applied separately. The insights, theory, and research from feminist psychoanalysis, somatic psychology and traumatology, and matricentric feminism have informed the main problem areas illustrated in Figure 4.2.

Psychological

- ◆ Focus on the problems of the lack of recognition of maternal embodied subjectivity and how this impacts mothers and the therapeutic relationship.
- ◆ Understanding how trauma impacts maternal embodied subjectivity and causes bodylessness and how claiming maternal embodied and relational subjectivity is crucial to the trauma healing process.

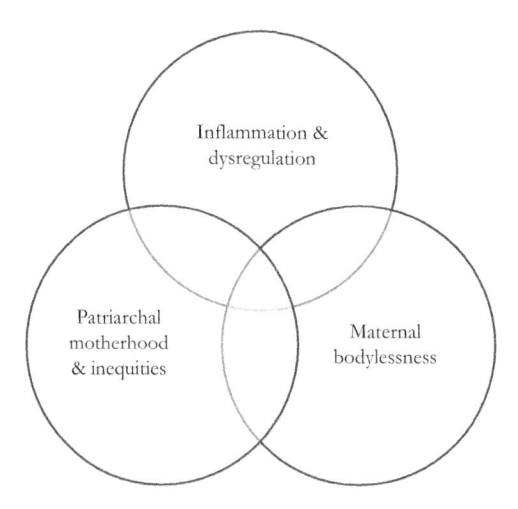

FIGURE 4.2 Main Problem Areas

- Appreciating that the maternal transition happens on experiential, somatic, unconscious, and nonverbal levels and narrative, cognitive, conscious, and verbal levels simultaneously, acknowledging their complex interplay.

Biological

- Appreciation of the coregulatory nature of our interpersonal biology and its salience in the perinatal period.
- Acknowledging both the vulnerabilities and the opportunities of the perinatal transition evidenced by research in psychoneuroimmunology, endocrinology, and maternal brain plasticity.
- Holistically anti-inflammatory support: Understanding of the role of perinatal stress and its links to depression and trauma and the importance of targeting inflammation.

Social

- Institutionalized and patriarchal motherhood, and intensive mothering ideologies impact Mental Health

and contribute to the disparities in Maternal Mental Health.
♦ Othering and discrimination related to maternal identity is an embodied experience that must be understood from a trauma perspective.
♦ Assertion of the diversity of maternal subjectivities through empowered or feminist mothering has a political activism potential. It is not limited to the individual realm but reaches into cultural and psychosocial discourses and community activism.

Treatment Goals and Strategy: Maternal Bodyfulness

The main problem (see Figure 4.2) informs the treatment goals. The overarching goal in *Somatic Maternal Healing* is:

To help the mother develop a mode of coregulation-supported somatically anchored reflections where she can mourn, play, process, and release traumatic memories so that she may eventually explore and synthesize the verbal and nonverbal and conscious and unconscious expressions of her maternal embodied and relational subjectivity. This is captured under the concept of maternal bodyfulness (see Figure 4.3). To balance the inherent vulnerability of the maternal transition with its potential for deeper healing of trauma on psychological, biological, and sociological levels, the treatment aims to support the mother in asserting her embodied subjectivity through maternal bodyfulness with:

1. Focus on supporting the assertion of maternal embodied subjectivity through the perinatal-specific coregulation mode of the therapeutic relationship, sensory awareness and vocabulary, and maternal body narrative and body identity.
2. Anti-inflammatory measures: Psychoeducation, stress reduction, referrals to health care providers to address inflammation-related issues like pain and auto-immune

```
                    Biological
               Target inflammation
               Interrupt stress cycles
               Nervous system
                  regulation
Psychological                          Social/Activism

Sensory awareness and                  Empowered mothering
    vocabulary                              Resisting
Body narrative and                       institutionalized
    identity                                motherhood


                    Maternal
                   Bodyfulness
```

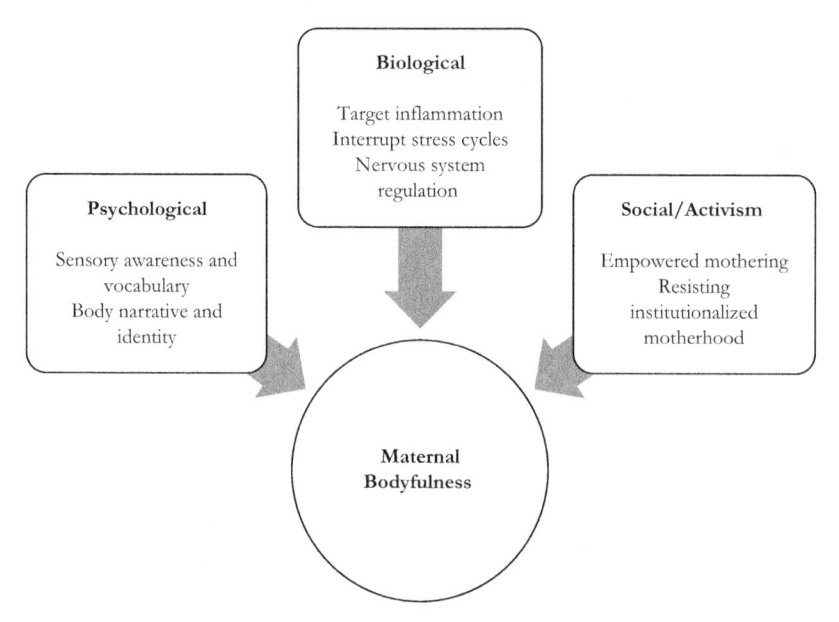

FIGURE 4.3 Maternal Bodyfulness

conditions, and nervous system somatic work for regulation and trauma resolution.
3. Cultivating empowered mothering and resistance against the oppression of institutionalized patriarchal motherhood.

The goal for the therapist in *Somatic Maternal Healing* is to build a capacity for *embodied* empathic attunement and work actively with somatic countertransferences specific to the perinatal transition. The ambition is for perinatal clinicians to build confidence in their work by anchoring their interventions on a foundation of somatic attunement that is highly sensitive to 1) the particular shifts of the maternal transition, 2) the clinician's countertransference reactions to these, 3) the manifestations of perinatal trauma, and 4) the coregulatory nature of the therapeutic relationship and daily life of mothering. Through the focus on the somatic relational aspects of perinatal work, clinicians work to increase their sensitivity to the nature of the maternal transition and the many layers of trauma in the perinatal period.

Key Clinical Skills

From the principles and treatment goals follow five essential clinical skills that will be the focus of Part II:

1. Ability to identify and track own patterns of nervous system activation.
2. Ability to identify and track clients' patterns of nervous system activation.
3. Familiarity with the particular forms of nervous system upheaval and dysregulation of the maternal transition.
4. Ability to actively use own somatic countertransference to deepen the therapeutic relationship, using knowledge about the landscape of the perinatal nervous system patterns and one's personal somatic biases.
5. Sensitivity to the client's verbal and nonverbal expressions of resisting (or seeking to resist) patriarchal motherhood and claiming embodied maternal subjectivity.

The therapist's ability to identify and track nervous system patterns in themselves and the client (Skills 1 and 2) are fundamental to somatic or body-oriented psychotherapy. They are also known as "body listening practices" (Caldwell, 2018b, p. 42). They are practiced through somatic attunement and resonance (see Chapter 5) and sensory awareness (see Chapter 6). They serve the purpose of establishing therapeutic safety and coregulation. They also aim to "sense the body in complex and non-judgmental ways" (Caldwell, 2018b, p. 42) and for the therapist to become an "interactive regulator" (Schore, 2021, p. 15). The landscape of the nervous system patterns of the maternal transition (Skill 3) is wide and cannot be exhaustively mapped since it intertwines with the nervous system manifestations of the client's individual trauma history. However, it is important for the clinician to develop knowledge of common perinatal somatic themes like the following:

- ♦ the evolution-based lowered survival reaction threshold that is activated relationally by the strong protective impulses of mothering an infant,

- reactions to the increase in dependency during the perinatal period,
- reactions to the bodily vulnerability and the significant body changes and shifts in body identity and body image of the maternal transition, and
- somatic reactions to the experience of maternal ambivalence (in its general form related to the baby but can also include ambivalence about the new mother self, the new maternal role and life, the new postpartum body and its body functions, the partner, or other family members).

The therapist must develop an awareness of how their biases related to the perinatal transition and its particular forms of dysregulation manifest *somatically* (Skill 4). Clinicians are widely trained to develop cognitive awareness of their biases and countertransference reactions, but mental awareness is not enough if the reactions cause somatic dysregulation in the therapist's nervous system that interferes with their ability to attune to the client. These dysregulation reactions occur in the therapist with or without their awareness. When clinicians have developed familiarity with the landscape of the perinatal nervous system patterns (Skill 3) and their somatic countertransference (Skill 4), they can intentionally self-regulate and actively use their reactions to enhance attunement and therapeutic safety.

Chapter 5 focuses on the attunement and resonance that are necessary for building the therapeutic alliance and relational safety that is the foundation for the new mother client to explore and express her embodied maternal subjectivity and subsequent trauma release. The clinician's awareness of the somatic aspects of their biases and countertransference reactions are foundational for cultivating sensitivity to the client's verbal and nonverbal expressions of resisting (or seeking to resist) institutionalized patriarchal motherhood and claiming embodied maternal subjectivity (Skill 5). Supporting the client's assertion of embodied maternal subjectivity begins with therapeutic safety, so barriers to somatic receptivity can be explored, including themes of bodylessness, and sensory awareness practices can be introduced

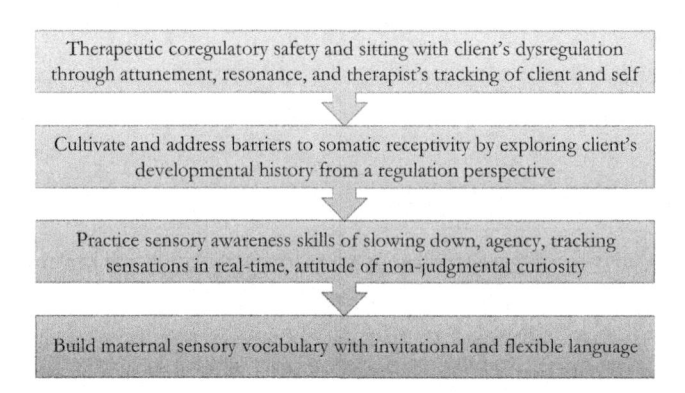

```
┌─────────────────────────────────────────────────────────────┐
│ Therapeutic coregulatory safety and sitting with client's   │
│ dysregulation through attunement, resonance, and            │
│ therapist's tracking of client and self                     │
└─────────────────────────────────────────────────────────────┘
                              ↓
┌─────────────────────────────────────────────────────────────┐
│ Cultivate and address barriers to somatic receptivity by    │
│ exploring client's developmental history from a regulation  │
│ perspective                                                 │
└─────────────────────────────────────────────────────────────┘
                              ↓
┌─────────────────────────────────────────────────────────────┐
│ Practice sensory awareness skills of slowing down, agency,  │
│ tracking sensations in real-time, attitude of non-judgmental│
│ curiosity                                                   │
└─────────────────────────────────────────────────────────────┘
                              ↓
┌─────────────────────────────────────────────────────────────┐
│ Build maternal sensory vocabulary with invitational and     │
│ flexible language                                           │
└─────────────────────────────────────────────────────────────┘
```

FIGURE 4.4 Therapeutic Phases of Building Maternal Sensory Awareness and Vocabulary

(see Figure 4.4). This will be unfolded in Chapter 6. A demonstration of how the principles and treatment goals translate into treatment planning will be provided in Chapter 8.

References

Borrell-Carrió, F., Suchman, A.L., & Epstein, R.M. (2004). The biopsychosocial model 25 years later: Principles, practice, and scientific inquiry. *Annals of Family Medicine, 2*(6), 576–582. 10.1370/afm.245

Caldwell, C.M. (2016) Body identity development: Definitions and discussions. *Body, Movement and Dance in Psychotherapy, 11*(4), 220–234. 10.1080/17432979.2016.1145141

Caldwell, C.M. (2018a). *Bodyfulness. Somatic practices for presence, empowerment, and waking up in this life*. Shambala Publications.

Caldwell, C.M. (2018b). Body identity development: Who we are and who we become. In C.M. Caldwell, & L.B. Leighton (Eds.), *Oppression and the body. Roots, resistance, and resolutions* (pp. 31–50). North Atlantic Books.

Levine, P.A. (2010). *In an unspoken voice. How the body releases trauma and restores goodness*. North Atlantic Books.

O'Reilly, A. (2021). *Matricentric feminism. Theory, activism, practice. The 2nd edition*. Demeter Press. 10.2307/j.ctv1k2j331

Schore, A.N. (2021). The interpersonal neurobiology of intersubjectivity. *Frontiers in Psychology, 12*, 648616. 10.3389/fpsyg.2021.648616

5

Working Somatically in the Perinatal Transferential Field

Attunement and Empathy in the Perinatal Context

Trust and safety are central factors in the somatic treatment of trauma (Kuhfuß et al., 2021). When we feel safe, we become open to connecting with others without feeling threatened (Porges, 2022). But can we just assume our usual safety-building clinical skills for the general population are appropriate when working with the perinatal client? The perinatal therapist must first and foremost be sensitive to the intense work of intersubjective nonverbal emotional communication that the mother is constantly engaged in with her baby. This means we attune differently to the perinatal client compared to other clients. Directing primary empathy and attention towards the coregulation aspect of mothering increases the trauma sensitivity of perinatal therapy by orienting the therapist towards regulation and its relational nature. As reviewed in Chapter 4, the attachment-building process is facilitated by the self-regulatory structures of the brain (Schore, 2012). This neurological development cannot be separated from the development of the entire body. The essence of somatically informed perinatal psychotherapy lies in the nonverbal affective *relational* dynamics that are sensitive to and welcoming of the body states of pregnancy, postpartum, and

DOI: 10.4324/9781003310914-8

mothering. These body states are characterized by fluid body boundaries, upheaval, expansion of subjectivity and the sense of self (see Chapter 1), massive endocrine shifts and neurobiological adaptations (see Chapter 2), pressures from cultural expectations (see Chapter 3), experiences of losses and uncertainty, and new forms of survival and protection responses.

The perinatal therapist must be empathic towards the maternal body states through non-verbal body-to-body attunement, making themselves available beyond an intellectual, reflective, and insight-oriented level. It is not enough to have a mental understanding of how pregnancy often entails severe fatigue, how breastfeeding can be a highly ambivalent experience, or how societal expectations for mothers are highly stressful and contradictory. *The perinatal therapist must be experienced in tracking their own somatic reactions to such knowledge and connecting this to their own nervous system history.* One of the most important forms of support in the perinatal period is to experience somatic attunement; to experience that the unique upheaval and dysregulation of one's maternal transition is received and experienced by a supportive other on not only a mental level but also – and especially – on a bodily level. A therapist's skills of embodied attunement are necessary for empowering a client to master self-regulation (Levine, 2010). We must offer the new mother an experience of being received on a bodily level, meaning that the wildness of her maternal transition is fully received, and not defended against, by the therapist. In this way, we listen to her in her raw embodied state, with our body.

When we acknowledge the somatic dimensions of perinatal therapy, we realize a whole range of struggles for the clinician of an experiential nature, which are not easily solved with mental analysis and intellectual efforts. It is crucial to adopt a mindset of primarily striving to attune before figuring out the mental state and meaning-makings of the client. A central clinical principle of the bottom-up approach is to value the struggles of attunement higher than the struggles of cognitive understanding. What this means is that we must struggle more to attune to our client's body and nervous system than we are struggling to figure out her mind or her cognitive activity. The new mother is experiencing constant intense bodily struggles to understand her baby's needs, and the therapist who also takes on the struggle to attune somatically can thereby mirror her state.

Being in the presence of a maternal body presents us with a nervous system situation unlike most other interactions in life. It is activating to witness a mother and her new maternal body in all the states of intense emotionality and dysregulation that arise in her work of mothering. It is common to get emotionally activated by the mere presence of a mother with a baby: The newborn's vulnerability elicits our deepest unconscious feelings of powerlessness. Mothers are subjected to the constant projections of that powerlessness from people around her as well as herself and her internalized beliefs. She is policed by her surroundings and polices herself. She is not a completely differentiated and independently functioning organism. The oscillations of her nervous system are intertwined with those of her baby. Positioning oneself as a therapist to a new mother involves an active engagement in this coregulatory dynamic. We are meant to be activated by this. From an affect regulation and somatic perspective, these reactions reflect the intensity of the coregulating field that anyone in the presence of the mother-infant pair is also biologically impacted by. They can also be considered from the feminist psychoanalytic perspective of the existential universal issue of acknowledging maternal embodied subjectivity reviewed in Chapter 1. The vicissitudes of perinatal nervous system functioning intertwine with cultural symbolic meanings and projections onto the maternal body that challenges our understanding of subjectivity. Attunement and empathy in perinatal therapy begins from this baseline of projection, activation, and dysregulation. The perinatal therapist must be acutely sensitive to these tensions that surround new mothers, including the therapist's own experience of and participation in them.

To help the client build awareness of and integrate her subjective experience for asserting her new embodied maternal subjectivity through maternal bodyfulness (see Chapters 3 and 6), we must first work with the foundation of how the self comes into experience through the intersubjective coregulating field of nonverbal interactions. Regulation cannot be separated from attachment and sense of self, as the attachment-building process and the development of the self-regulatory structures of the brain are intertwined and mutually dependent (Schore, 2012). The interactions between two people become emotionally meaningful because their exchanges have a regulatory purpose (Hill, 2015; Schore, 2021). It is when we attune to the psychobiological landscape of the perinatal period that we can form an effective and meaningful therapeutic relationship with the new mother. The perinatal therapist engages with this landscape through resonance, a term widely used in body-centered psychotherapy (LaPierre, 2015; Selvam, 2022).

Resonance and the New Mother

Levine (2010) states that it is crucial that clinicians don't protect themselves against their clients' sensations and feelings because it is through this somatic attunement that we can establish the relational relative safety that is needed for intersubjective regulation and ultimately the release of the nervous system patterns of immobility and fear responses that heals trauma. This means we must be willing and available to experience our clients' states in our own bodies. Resonance is the therapist's powerful instrument for attunement and connecting, indeed the basis of intimate relationships (Levine, 2010; Selvam, 2022). It is the active therapeutic use of feeling into the client's state using one's own nervous system and sensory awareness. In this way, it also becomes a diagnostic tool (LaPierre, 2015). We attune to our clients through resonance to help them regulate and embody their emotions (Selvam, 2021). LaPierre (2015) describes resonance as "transmission of sensations, visceral reactions, emotions, images, and thoughts from one person to another" (p. 21). In somatically attuned therapy, we communicate to our clients that our bodily presence is available to the client (Orbach, 2006). This attitude is at the center of resonance: The therapist communicates that their nervous system is available. Resonance is effectively the therapist's capacity for what Schore has described as "interpersonal brain synchronization" (2021). It begins with the integrative use of two key clinical skills, tracking one's own and the client's nervous system. A common technique in body psychotherapy to enhance attunement is to resonate with a client's state by mirroring their vocal, facial, and other body expressions (Selvam, 2021). This can also be used reversely, when the therapist limits the mirroring to reduce overwhelm from too intense resonance. With balanced resonance, the therapist becomes an "interactive regulator" (Schore, 2021) to the client. When we feel what our client is experiencing in their body with our own body and then regulate ourselves, directly impacting the intersubjective field of coregulation, we are using resonance to help the client regulate (Selvam, 2021). Perinatal therapists must have a developed relationship with their own embodiment and sensory awareness if they are to somatically attune and resonate effectively.

Resonance is important in the therapeutic relationship because it facilitates repair. When there are ruptures in the therapeutic relationship that we cannot immediately or appropriately repair verbally, we are still able to work towards repair on a nonverbal level by returning to the foundational regulating skills. Feeling into the client's somatic experience of the rupture allows the therapist to demonstrate a non-defensive attitude and maintain a commitment to coregulation. The therapist tracks the somatic impact of the rupture on both the client and themselves and works to repair it nonverbally by returning to synchronicity with resonance and affect attunement. The new mother is constantly doing micro-repairs with her baby that are nonverbal and characterized by synchronization and contingent responsivity (Beebe & Lachmann, 1988; Schore, 2021). The coregulation that comes from the therapist's embodied attunement to the client is founded on this developmental nonverbal dynamic of the early infant-caregiver relationship, which is the basis of attachment formation. The experiences of valuable repairs often don't become "official" in the therapeutic conversation through verbalization, but they are still experienced somatically by the therapist and client. Some therapists are taught that repair is only valid if it is concretely verbalized in the therapeutic conversation. This is unfortunate, as the nonverbal experience of relational repair through resonance is deeply healing and a primary experiential condition of the perinatal period. It is also especially important for trauma survivors because their suffering is connected to the way their engagement in nonverbal coregulation has been impacted by trauma.

How Trauma Impacts Perinatal Coregulation

Affect dysregulation lies at the core of all psychopathology (Schore, 2012), including the range of symptoms that stem from trauma. The affect regulation model is built on the conceptualization of trauma as the key factor in an individual's development and life-long mental health through the way it impacts regulation. Childhood maltreatment, also called developmental trauma, manifests in adult life as dysregulation issues. Many survivors of developmental trauma might not present as if they have lived a life deeply impacted by dysregulation. This is due to the resilience and a range of comprehensive compensation strategies that enable trauma survivors to for example hold a job and maintain relationships despite daily struggles with dysregulation, which takes a toll on their health. The perinatal transition can unearth a new mother's developmental trauma to the surprise of herself and her surroundings. This type of underlying trauma, which a woman may or may not have had awareness of, manifests in the coregulation with her baby and those around her. New mothers have different levels of detectable depression, anxiety, trauma, and stress disorders which are assessed as part of the normal standard of care, but the focus of the trauma-responsive perinatal therapist, especially in the initial interactions of building rapport, should be to assess the woman's current self-regulation and coregulation functioning as well as her regulation history, which is directly connected to relational functioning. Assessing the correct diagnosis is important for proper treatment planning, but this diagnosis is useless without the context of trauma history in the sense of how it has and is concretely impacting a client's regulation and relational functioning.

People with a trauma history often perceive neutral stimuli as threatening. The new mother with a trauma history is further challenged as the question of safety is made complex by her appropriate impulses to protect her baby. She may understand rationally that the lactation consultant entering the room is not an actual threat, but if conflicts arise where she feels dismissed and there isn't adequate attunement in their interaction, her nervous system will respond with a survival-based reaction for both her own protection and her baby's. The maternal transition makes the new mother hypervigilant for adaptive reasons. The new mother with a trauma history will often experience the hypervigilance becoming so overwhelming that it interferes with her ability to take in attunement and relational support during a time when she is acutely dependent on it. A vicious cycle can occur where a mother's anxiety increases as she experiences a lack of relational support, which exacerbates her feelings of threat, causing her to withdraw or be guarded in her interaction with others, making it less likely for her to have experiences of attunement. In polyvagal theory, the bodily state related to trauma (dorsal vagal) is characterized by a disengagement from the social engagement system (ventral vagal) (Porges, 2022). The attuned perinatal therapist works to break this cycle, firstly by assessing the mother's experience and perception of her surroundings and whether she feels attuned to them. The therapist must adjust their expectations for the nonverbal aspects of interaction for this assessment if they are to help the client back to social engagement through relational safety.

It is essential to acknowledge that general perinatal hypervigilance is not only common but also biologically appropriate. This is done both indirectly through the therapist's nonverbal attitude and directly through psychoeducational statements that normalize and empathize with perinatal overwhelm. As the client's trauma history is assessed, the therapist can also normalize the added layers of dysregulation given the client's history. Therapists should not underestimate the importance of psychoeducational reflective feedback to the effect of *"It is very understandable how the hospital stay was difficult for you and gave you anxiety given what you have told me about your experiences with surgeries"* or *"It makes a lot of sense that you feel very scared about even thinking about breastfeeding given what you have told me about your experiences of having your body boundaries disrespected"*. When statements like these are given within the context of embodied attunement and resonance, they can help clients build the capacity for reflecting on themselves as humans impacted by traumatic experiences as opposed to internalizing their trauma response as an absolute value statement about their character, a common trauma response.

Coregulation and Shame

The landscape of the maternal transition is riddled with potential trauma themes that primarily manifest somatically and relationally. A central theme of trauma is shame, especially in relation to intergenerational trauma, which is commonly activated by the maternal transition because it is a deeply visceral and somatic lifecycle transition in the female lifespan where a woman is brought into the maternal lineage of her ancestral chain through a bodily event. Shame is notoriously hard to process and work with therapeutically because it originates in preverbal body states (Schore, 1998). It is often strongly coupled with body themes that abound in the maternal transition, for example, feeling dysregulated and rejected because of it, or feeling bodily fragmented and fearful of being judged for it. The shame state is characterized by a shutting down of the social engagement system. Shame is a right-brain relationally based feeling and therefore directly related to the early relational coregulation functions, specifically attachment transactions involving misattuned face-to-face interactions (Schore, 1998). Relationally, shame reactions are often not only about feeling rejected by the other, but also about wanting to protect the other from oneself. The self is experienced as bad or even toxic and unworthy of receiving care from others. Somatically this means that one's body state is experienced as a threat to the other and must therefore be held back from the intersubjective coregulation field, as a survival response. If a therapist struggles to feel anything from the client, it can be a sign of the client dealing with the loss of sensation or dissociation, but can it also be about the shame that is making them withhold themselves from the intersubjective field to "protect" the therapist (Selvam, 2021). Shame states that impact the somatic intersubjective field can also be intertwined with what Orbach (2006) has described as a lack of the sense of being embodied. Attachment trauma can manifest somatically in this way because the lack of caregiver attunement caused a halting of the client's development of their sense of being embodied. When the new mother who carries the trauma of a lacking sense of embodiment is thrown into the task of being the steward of her baby's emerging sense of a bodily self, her own trauma materializes in an unprecedented way.

Shame dynamics are complex in the perinatal period because of the mother's necessary narcissistic investment in her baby manifesting in the fluidity of body boundaries (see Chapter 1). The mother's shame about herself is therefore often intertwined with her ambivalent feelings towards her baby. A common theme in perinatal therapy is a mother's worries about her baby being "difficult", to herself or the surroundings, which she might take on, as if her baby's impact on others is her responsibility. Other common shame-related themes are narratives of the "failures" of the maternal body in relation to reproductive functions, a form of maternal bodylessness. Mothers often express frustration and despair related to feeling that their bodies "failed" them or failed at living up to expectations for successful reproductive or maternal functioning. Maternal body failure narratives are often related to shame dynamics and maternal bodylessness (see Chapter 3).

Key Clinical Skill of Somatic Attunement and Resonance

There are four key clinical skills that facilitate somatic attunement and resonance when working in the perinatal period:

- ◆ Ability to identify and track your own patterns of nervous system activation.

- Ability to identify and track your client's patterns of nervous system activation.
- Familiarity with the particular forms of nervous system upheaval and dysregulation of the perinatal transition.
- Active use of somatic countertransference to deepen the therapeutic relationship, using knowledge about the landscape of the perinatal nervous system patterns and one's personal somatic biases.

These skills are applied simultaneously, but they are learned and practiced by the therapist in this order. The therapist's own tracking of their nervous system activity is foundational to attunement and resonance. When the therapist has built the skills of tracking, learned to use sensations to feel into the client's state (resonance), developed familiarity of the landscape of the perinatal nervous system patterns, and identified their personal somatic biases and reaction patterns specific to the perinatal field, they can begin to actively work with somatic countertransference to deepen the therapeutic work relationally. The fifth skill of sensitivity to the client's verbal and nonverbal expressions of resisting institutionalized motherhood and how they are claiming embodied maternal subjectivity through sensory vocabulary will be addressed in Chapter 6.

The perinatal nervous system landscape includes (but is not limited to): A lowered survival reaction threshold that is mediated relationally due to the protective instincts, reactions to the significant increase in dependency, reactions to the increased body vulnerability and the significant shifts in body identity and body image, reactions to new states of intense ambivalence, and new forms of sensory coregulatory pleasure. Maternal ambivalence usually refers to a mother's feelings about her baby, but it can also include ambivalence about the new mother self, the new maternal role and life, the new postpartum body and its body functions, the partner, or other family members. The perinatal therapist must develop knowledge of their own biases related to the perinatal transition and its particular forms of dysregulation, and specifically how these biases manifest *somatically*. It is good for clinicians to have a cognitive awareness of their personal feelings and beliefs about maternal themes, but a mental awareness of this is not enough to address the *somatic* aspects of this countertransference, especially any dysregulation that interferes with the clinician's ability to attune. It is possible to reject, ignore, or otherwise defend against the somatic aspects of the transferential field, but it is not possible to *not* be affected by perinatal resonance dynamics when doing psychotherapy with a perinatal client.

Nervous System Tracking

Practicing the ability to track sensations is a continuation of the ordinary developmental task of gradually learning to interpret interoceptive information that all humans go through (Levine, 2010). Our individual relationship with sensory awareness is reflective of our developmental history. The maturation of the nervous system is facilitated by body-to-body coregulation (Levine et al., 2018; Schore, 2021). The attuned perinatal therapist is therefore indirectly assessing the client's relational and trauma history as part of the nervous system tracking. The practice of tracking has a regulatory effect in itself (Selvam, 2021). It is from observation of the client's subtle nervous system shifts that the therapist can offer feedback that helps the client build sensory awareness (Levine, 2010). Since awareness of sensations is foundational to regulation, the sensory awareness that builds from tracking the nervous system is a central resource. As reviewed in Chapter 4, regulation forms from relational experiences of nervous system synchronization. Nervous system tracking can therefore be understood as a concretization of the coregulatory relationship building. The therapist and client cocreate "rhythms of being together" as manifestations of the therapeutic relationship (Carroll, 2014, p. 20). Good attunement comes from tracking the subtlest actions and states in others (Caldwell, 2018a). It is important for the therapist to notice sudden shifts in both the client and themselves. Especially the latter can indicate important resonance dynamics (Selvam, 2021). Tracking themselves and the client enables the therapist to track the relational process (Carroll, 2014). When the therapist offers the foundational coregulation of tracking the nervous system of the therapeutic dyad, they facilitate the client's building of sensory awareness. The emphasis should be on the client's experience of the *shifts* in their internal state, as the felt experience of nervous system shifts is central to regulation (Levine et al., 2018). It is also through the awareness of how sensations shift that clients learn the transitory nature of dysregulation and overwhelm (Levine, 2010).

Sensations can be categorized into interoception, exteroception, and proprioception (Caldwell, 2018a). Interoception, or the "felt sense", is the sensory data of our internal bodily state (Levine, 2010) such as respiration, muscle tension, temperature changes, thirst, and blood flow. Exteroception refers to our sensory input from our direct surroundings through our five senses (Caldwell, 2018a), also called "orienting" (Levine, 2010). Proprioception is our sensations related to movement, posture, and spatial orientation (Caldwell, 2018a), in other words, the brain's registration of bodily movement in time and space (Carroll, 2014). Clients are often not aware of the differences between interoceptive, exteroceptive, and proprioceptive shifts. Nervous system tracking as a therapeutic tool involves comprehensive psychoeducation that becomes coregulatory when done with a nonjudgmental, exploratory, invitational, and supportive attitude. In somatic therapy, the client is guided to bring their attention to interoceptive and proprioceptive experiences and to orient to their surroundings through their senses (Payne et al., 2015). The client's subjective experience is valued and serves as the starting point for exploration. Tracking nervous system activity is also called "body listening practices" (Caldwell, 2018b, p. 42). This description is helpful to emphasize that the focus of sensory tracking should be the therapist and client listening to the client's body states, as collaborators. "Listening" to the body consists of the conscious tracking of "shifts in gut feelings, breath, heart rate, and bracing patterns" in both client and therapist (LaPierre, 2015, p. 15). The therapist observes and monitors the client's nervous system activation patterns and elicits and attends to the client's self-report of interoceptive shift (Levine et al., 2018).

The client's emotional expressions, postural shifts and gestures, and autonomic nervous system shifts can be directly observed. The therapist tracks whether the client is becoming more or less organized and regulated as a result of the "shifts that arise from present-tense alterations in patterns of attention" (Levine et al., 2018, p. 620). Tracking is procedural and "often fast, complex, and intricate" (Carroll, 2014, p. 17).

When practicing nervous system tracking, client self-report requires psychoeducational invitations: The therapist explains the importance of the client's internal experiences to the therapeutic process and uses invitational language to support the client in expressing and describing their sensations. It is crucial to acknowledge the limitations of language when trying to capture experiences of a nonverbal nature. Encouraging the client to slow down their movements and reflections helps them orient to their proprioceptive level of experience (Levine et al., 2018). The phenomenological awareness of nervous system tracking requires slowing down (Carroll, 2014). When the therapeutic relationship is established and the therapist has gained knowledge of the client's state, they can begin to gently orient the client towards stabilizing sensations, thereby facilitating regulatory support. The principle of slowing down when tracking sensations will be further elaborated in Chapter 6.

Some individuals, often trauma survivors, are easily overwhelmed when tracking interoceptive information because early in their development they learned to associate bodily sensations with danger as a self-protective defense in response to lack of coregulation from their caregivers (Johnson, 2021; Levine, 2010). Paradoxically, it is also a common symptom of trauma to be drawn towards the interoceptive overwhelm of dysregulation and traumatic memories (Levine et al., 2018). When tracking of interoception is overwhelming, clients should be helped to orient towards their external environment (exteroception) and proprioception. Orienting to the external environment is a central resource to facilitate regulation (Johnson, 2021; Levine, 2010). The therapist supports the client in recognizing this pattern and identifying resources related to exteroception, to balance this impulse of focusing on dysregulation. As the therapist is working with the client to recognize this pattern and identify the resources to counter the overwhelm from it, it is crucial that the therapist does not dismiss the client's experience of overwhelm or convey a message of rush to get the client out of it. The therapist must first attune to the client's dysregulation to facilitate any changes to it. The therapist supports the client in discovering a sense of mastery and agency when directing their attention back and forth between internal sensations and the environment. This element of agency will be elaborated in Chapter 6.

Sitting with the Dysregulation of the Perinatal Period

The intersubjective therapeutic space of perinatal work will often involve high levels of dysregulation. This is not only due to the high prevalence of PMADs and perinatal trauma, but also because of the adaptations of reproduction that impact the activation threshold of the new mother's nervous system. The survival response system is both heightened and complicated by the relational component of the caregiving situation: The new mother experiences a heightened sense of existential vulnerability and need to activate survival responses that are not only about the survival of her own organism. It is not possible to locate an absolute demarcation line between the normal adaptive evolution-based activation of the new mother's nervous system and trauma- and stress-related reactions.

The depth of the grief and loss in perinatal trauma can elicit an urge in clinicians to seek out immediate meaning-making to soothe the client. The somatic approach to sitting with dysregulation means that the clinician does not focus solely on helping the client arrive at mental solutions, but instead works with resonance to establish a felt experience of being together. The aim is that the client experiences their grief and dysregulation as a bodily state that can be contained in the therapeutic relationship. Whatever the content of the dysregulation, the therapist is first sitting with it rather than interpreting it (Orbach, 2006). Holding space for the new mother's dysregulation means we must consciously suspend our eagerness to get her to a place of regulation and calmness. The goal is to eventually facilitate regulation and grounding, but it is crucial to not skip over the first step of attuning to her dysregulation. That step is vulnerable to the archaic experiences of being dismissed, shut off, resented, or rejected by the other upon whom one is deeply dependent. It is also trauma's litmus test of the therapeutic relationship. It is a significant advantage of somatic modalities that the therapist is resourced to regulate themselves when experiencing the client's intense dysregulation in the transferential field (Leddick, 2018).

As reviewed in Chapter 4, the developmental foundation of a mother's self-regulation is her early life experiences of having her own dysregulation attuned and responded to by her caregiver through their capacity for self- and coregulation. As the new mother is immersed in the task of tolerating both her own and her baby's dysregulation, her life experiences of how others have tolerated and reacted to her dysregulation are reflected in her embodied experience of the coregulating relationship with her baby. Perinatal therapy means we enter this field of Matryoshka dolls of coregulation. The starting point must therefore be to sit fully with the dysregulation. As long as the implicit message of the therapist's physical presence in the room is not one of acknowledgment of her dysregulation and willingness to be impacted by the therapeutic relationship, her nervous system will not move towards connection and integration. Selvam (2021) points out that therapists who are not used to feeling their bodies will understandably struggle with sensing the dysregulation of their clients through resonance. This is a concern in perinatal therapy too, especially for therapists who believe they must be perfectly regulated.

The perinatal therapist does not need – in fact, should *not* – attempt to achieve a state of perfect self-regulation to effectively attune to perinatal dysregulation. By tracking their own nervous system and working in the resonance of feeling into the client's distress, the therapist is balancing attunement to dysregulation while keeping "one foot anchored" in their own sensory awareness to stay regulated (Selvam, 2021). This mirrors the mother's work of coregulating with her baby by feeling the baby's distress while self-regulating in the service of both. When practicing these clinical skills, the therapist must work to normalize their own dysregulation and discomfort and appreciate the healing functions of it the therapeutic relationship. Any urges to eliminate the discomfort of dysregulation that the therapist has due to their own trauma should be identified through nervous system tracking and self-reflection. Selvam (2021) states the therapist should work to resonate with the client's dysregulation by setting a clear intention to welcome it and then to self-regulate enough to make the experience bearable, but not so much that the resonant relationship is compromised. The therapist can self-regulate by bringing gentle awareness to sensations during the session.

Examples of therapist self-regulation tools:

♦ Track sensations related to gravity and feeling anchored in the chair.
♦ Use unnoticeable self-touch like a hand on the knee or folding hands or any point of contact between body parts and focus on the sensations of making contact.
♦ Locate the most stable sensation internally and maintain awareness of it.

The therapist must resonate with flexibility, meaning they are mindful that they can at times be inaccurate or not elicit the desired positive response from the client (Selvam, 2021). This balance is challenging, especially when working with perinatal clients who have suffered intense and multiple forms of trauma. It can be helpful to keep a continued focus on the purposes of balanced resonance with the client's dysregulation: To facilitate the client's experience of being attuned to, to break the vicious cycle of withdrawal caused by trauma, and to help the client move towards a bodily state of receptivity; the foundation for trauma healing.

Somatic Receptivity

Parenting is about giving and caring. But pregnancy, delivery, and postpartum also involve a lot of receiving. Going through the maternal transition is a vulnerable developmental period that elicits concrete needs for care and subsequent vulnerability. Not just the obvious needs for obstetric and prenatal care, but also emotional and relational care – and their somatic components; the corresponding bodily states of receiving. The new mother's nervous system requires care: Her nervous system is newborn in the sense of the upgrade, expansion, and transformation that having a baby will do to her body – and must be cared for and responded to from that perspective. Caring for a newborn requires relating deeply to the somatic states of vulnerability and dependency of that first stage of life. Bonding with a newborn is a nonverbal and visceral experience involving intense identification with and mirroring the state of purely receiving. It is emotionally hard (and sometimes impossible) to hold and nurture a baby with your body (the only way you *can* hold and nurture a baby) if you are disconnected from the sensations and states of being held and nurtured yourself. Holding and nurturing require a particular openness in the nervous system. Therefore, the somatic elements of psychotherapy with the pregnant or new mother must be practiced with an emphasis on cultivating receptivity.

Somatic receptivity is about building a relationship with the felt experience of receiving. The ability to receive support through coregulation requires a connection to the felt experience of sensations. The many factors that cause bodylessness (see Chapter 3) influence a person's relationship with receiving. The sensations of receiving, being held and nurtured, and the feelings associated with it are important to explore, expand, and practice collaboratively in the therapeutic relationship. This work brings up a challenge that intersects the micro/individual level with the macro/psychosocial: Somatic receptivity is particularly hard for expecting and new mothers because women are largely socialized to prioritize giving more than receiving. As discussed in Chapter 3, gender role expectations for mothers are steeped in the valorization of giving and self-sacrifice through intensive mothering ideology, causing the particular form of bodylessness that impact mothers. The expectations for mothers through cultural discourse are so self-effacing that many new mothers express intense guilt about receiving anything. The very experience of receiving can feel unsafe or activating for the new mother, especially in the context of relational trauma. As clinicians, we can psychoeducate thoroughly on the importance of self-care, and yet our clients will report intense struggles, guilt, and overwhelm which reflects the cultural pressures and expectations of patriarchal motherhood and the lack of somatic receptivity that this cultural pressure causes. New mothers will often fully agree on a rational level with our psychoeducation on the importance of getting their needs met too. But if their nervous systems never developed this capacity or were taught to shut down any states of receptivity, they will not be readily able to receive support on a somatic level from family or professionals. This barrier is even more exacerbated for trauma survivors who experience a profound disconnect from the body. Healing requires receiving. Cognitive insights are not enough when learning to receive; it also requires discovery and practicing of the felt experience of somatic receptivity.

How Trauma Interferes with Somatic Receptivity

A wide range of conditions can interfere with the new mother's somatic receptivity. From a trauma perspective, the primary reason for the lack of somatic receptivity is self-protective guardedness. Safety is a prerequisite for engaging in social interactions that have coregulatory capacities (Porges, 2022). The physical state of hypervigilance is the opposite of the physical state of receptivity, which is characterized by social engagement and safety. Without adequate safety, we cannot engage in the coregulation states that receiving requires. The practical realities of caring for an infant make for a state of constant giving if the new mother doesn't have adequate family support and/or has trauma- or stress-induced hypervigilance.

More than anything, trauma impacts our ability to receive support through embodied attunement and coregulation.

Attachment trauma causes a tendency to be watchful for what about oneself is received and what is rejected (Orbach, 2009). The client who suffered abuse experienced that being open to receiving was unsafe. A mother with a tendency to be wary about her wishes or patterns of nonverbal neediness might be flooded with anxiety from the wave of neediness of her postpartum body and situation and the reactivation of developmental trauma it causes. If having needs or experiences of being cared for (nonverbally and somatically) were imbued with negativity in her family of origin dynamics, the new demands of the postpartum period will likely be experienced as brutal and frustrating. Receiving becomes a particularly vulnerable experience in the perinatal period, where intimate body functions and needs are undergoing intense changes. This is closely related to the previously mentioned dynamics of shame that impact the capacity for coregulatory engagement and imbue the experience of receiving with a feeling of threat. The cognitive correlates of the bodily shame state are often negative core beliefs about self, for example, feeling unworthy of receiving or fears that opening oneself to receiving will cause one to "lose control" and be overwhelmed by neediness and longings. The perinatal period challenges and changes a woman's entire system of dependency and having her needs met. Everything from physical and practical needs to needs for emotional connection and spiritual guidance change as the mother and family adjust to the needs of the baby. A new mother's needs are often unpredictable and hard to figure out, which can elicit fear of the unknown, especially the sudden needs of the pregnant or postpartum body. The bodily needs of pregnancy, delivery, postpartum recovery, and new motherhood intertwine with the new emotional needs, and the needs of the baby and other family members. The experience of unmet needs is, for many mothers, difficult to articulate – especially if it activates trauma memories.

It is not only negative experiences with receiving that impact somatic receptivity. Lack of embodied experience of receiving contributes to a person's nervous system forming in ways that do not include experiences of receiving physical attunement. This can be the case in individuals who only experienced receiving in the form of money, goods, or other transactions, that were not somatically anchored. Cultural dynamics also impact new mothers' somatic receptivity. The idea of receiving as primarily a commercialized commodity that must convey status can form unconscious beliefs and interfere with the development of somatic patterns related to receiving. Gender role expectations, family dynamics, and cultural values play a part in this. Systemic conditions related to lack of resources, direct poverty, discrimination, and high levels of stress also impact an individual's relationship with receiving.

When we emphasize somatic attunement over cognitive understanding and feel into the experience of the client through resonance, the aim is to support the client in cultivating somatic receptivity; their capacity for bodily states that allow for taking in coregulatory support. Like we, directly and indirectly, offer psychoeducational acknowledgment of the new mother's perinatal dysregulation, we also work nonverbally and verbally with somatic receptivity to help her build awareness of the *somatic* aspects of her needs, her experience of getting them met, and how her developmental history impacts this. Therapists commonly explore the topic of needs and self-care with clients with the intention of empowering the client to identify effective strategies for getting their needs met. If this theme is explored from a mental and practical perspective without attention to the somatic aspects of how the client physically experiences receiving support and attunement, the client's foundation for taking anything in might be missed. A key aspect here is the client's experience of safety. If a therapist has spent several sessions exploring self-care with a client who expresses frustrations about the efforts not helping her feel better, her experience of somatic receptivity could be a missing factor to explore. Ideally, the therapist will use the client's experience of support in the sessions as a starting point for this. Tracking of the nervous system shifts of the therapeutic dyad is central information for the therapist's assessment of the client's experience of somatic receptivity. A new mother's somatic receptivity is explored through the somatic oscillations of co-regulation in the therapeutic dyad. When the client's relationship with somatic receptivity is assessed and explored by the therapeutic dyad, barriers can be targeted by the therapist's active use of somatic countertransference.

Somatic Countertransference

Where resonance is the therapist's active use of empathizing and relating to the client by feeling into the body state using their own body and sensations (Selvam, 2021), countertransference is widely understood as the therapist's unconscious or conscious reactions to the client and the client's transference based on the therapist's own psychology. Although the phenomenon of resonance is ubiquitous – that humans are impacted by each other's feelings on a bodily level (LaPierre, 2015) – resonance in the therapy setting is the active use of sensory awareness and embodied attunement to cultivate relationship-building empathy with the client. LaPierre (2015) argues that tracking the body indeed helps the therapist distinguish between countertransference in the sense of their own subjective experiences and responses that are driven by somatic empathy (i.e., resonance) with the client. When therapists are trained in using sensory awareness and resonance, they are better equipped at addressing the somatic aspects of their countertransference. This opens the potential for using it to deepen the therapeutic work. When the somatic dynamics of the transferential field are acknowledged as instrumental to the therapeutic relationship, the goal of treatment is expanded to include the development and healing of the client's embodied sense of self. In this way, somatic countertransference is not only symptoms of dysregulation to be "fixed", nor is it only clinical information to analyze; it is part of the intersubjective co-creation of the felt experience of being an embodied self that an attuned therapeutic relationship consists of. Orbach (2006) describes the importance of scrutinizing one's somatic reactions in the therapy room. The body becomes "a stethoscope-like instrument" (Orbach, 2009, p. 63) for listening to the client. Attending to the somatic aspects of countertransference facilitates somatic receptivity in the client. How we receive our clients' bodies is crucial for how they can experience somatic receptivity internally.

A relational approach to the development and disturbances of body image must be reflected in a therapeutic technique focusing on awareness of bodily feelings states in the transference-countertransference (Orbach, 2006, 2009). Working somatically in the transferential field requires a focus on shared psycho-sensory experience (Harrang et al., 2022). We must apply this attentiveness to the bodily relationality of our work. Orbach states that she examines her countertransference and "the corporeal intersubjectivity" (2006, p. 97). The aim of this is to understand the body's subjectivity and intersubjectivity and register how the body is present in countertransference. When the therapist is open to the somatic layers of countertransference, the therapist's body can receive and embody the "body-to-body relational mismatching" of the client's intersubjective history (Orbach, 2006, p. 100). A greater capacity for conflicting feelings is central to affect tolerance in intersubjective psychoanalysis (Selvam, 2021). The clinician's tolerance of conflictual feelings is expanded by attentiveness to the somatic countertransference. When the transferential field is acknowledged and appreciated as a realm of somatic dynamics, countertransference can be made use of in the service of supporting the mother's assertion of her new subjectivity, in other words, her maternal bodyfulness.

Orbach (2006) contends we must help our clients to *have* bodies. Working experientially and relationally towards experiencing an embodied sense of self is not only crucial for trauma treatment, but also carries an added layer of challenge due to the ontological and intersubjective challenge of maternal embodied subjectivity discussed in Chapter 1. How do we help our clients transition into having and being *maternal* bodies? This requires the therapist to firstly accept and tolerate the dysregulation coming from the two-fold upheaval of the sense of self that the maternal transition and trauma cause, and secondly to make active use of the transferential field in a somatic way to facilitate the client's relational discovery of being embodied. Working with the client towards discovering, verbalizing, and expressing the new maternal bodily self cannot be rushed or forced without adequate relational work of attunement to the perinatal dysregulation through resonance. It is not simply attuning to emotional distress or sympathetic arousal; it is to resonate with the existential destabilization of the sense of being an embodied and clearly defined subject. For a new mother with developmental trauma, we must start from a place of welcoming her experiences of having internalized negativity towards her body, being a fragmented bodily self, or lack of experience of having a body at all, and how all of these feelings are exacerbated by mothering. Successful trauma treatment will therefore change the client's relationship with herself, her embodiment, her embodied relationships with others, and how these intertwine.

The common phrase that "when a baby is born, so is a mother" not only points to the understanding of the new maternal role added to the mother's identity. From a somatic perspective, the maternal transition brings a woman back to the ontological realm of arriving into one's subjectivity through the body from which we all begin life (what Orbach (2006) calls the preintegrated body). The nature of mothering makes it challenging to achieve coherence in one's maternal body narrative. Many new mothers experience a process of grieving the body they never had or the bodily experiences they never had, as they experience the demands of fulfilling their babies' needs for embodied attunement. The unique vulnerability of the postpartum experience activates losses of never having experienced full containment of one's most vulnerable states. It is a deep grief to work through on a bodily non-verbal level. We must first work to establish body coherence (Orbach, 2006) before we can build a body narrative (Caldwell, 2016) and from that develop a bodyfully anchored sense of self (Caldwell, 2018a, 2018b). Body narrative and maternal bodyfulness will be addressed in Chapter 6.

Somatic Attunement and Resonance in Perinatal Telehealth

Telehealth offers some unique advantages specific to the postpartum client who might be in the hospital or at home with her baby. Telehealth increases accessibility to specialized perinatal mental health care, including in rural areas that tend to be underserved (Wassef & Wassef, 2022). The added overwhelm of the logistics of traveling to an office with an infant, especially in the early postpartum phase of recovery, is a significant barrier to treatment for many new mothers. Throughout the first year postpartum, new mothers have several medical appointments, both for their own follow-up care and child visits with pediatricians. This can be a source of significant stress, especially for the new mother suffering from PMADs or trauma reactions. Wassef and Wassef (2022) note that because perinatal women are at higher risk of not receiving treatment, the increase in accessibility may be the largest benefit of the shift to telemedicine for this population. A systematic review and meta-analysis by Zhao and colleagues (2021) of the efficacy of telehealth prior to the pandemic found a reduction in symptoms in women with PPD. Another study by Ackerman and colleagues (2021) demonstrated client satisfaction for perinatal women receiving mental health services via telehealth. Furthermore, one study showed that telehealth implementation for postpartum care during the COVID-19 pandemic was associated with decreased racial disparities in postpartum visit attendance (Kumar et al., 2022). While these studies are promising, the results must be weighed against the missed benefits of in-person treatment, which has been a key intervention in perinatal mental health to address the social isolation of mothering (Wassef & Wassef, 2022). Perinatal therapists must also consider the preferences, needs, and trauma history of the individual client, who might benefit more from in-person therapy.

The post-pandemic realities of online therapy bring challenges to attuned trauma therapy that focuses on coregulation. Aligned with the principle of trustworthiness and transparency in trauma-informed care (Polmanteer et al., 2019), perinatal therapists should explain the advantages and limitations of telehealth. Openness about both advantages and disadvantages of the treatment form is part of the informed consent process that can foster reflection on the client's needs and goals for treatment. While the limitations of coregulation through telehealth should not be underestimated, neither should we underestimate the potential for attuning through resonance when providing therapy online. Selvam (2021) has pointed out how it is possible to provide attuned therapy online namely by active use of resonance. It then becomes acutely important to actively work with tracking one's own nervous system and resonating with the client using one's own body. When tracking the client in online work, therapists must pay close attention to tone of voice, facial gestures, and body postures, and must therefore work with the client to optimize the level of technical accessibility for this. Online therapy offers the therapist an opportunity to observe some of the client's real-life environment (Wassef & Wassef, 2022). This can be used to deepen the resonance and when working with the client to explore their self-regulation circumstances and practices. Exercises meant to help the client practice their sensory awareness in their daily life, for example during caregiving tasks that make up a significant portion of new mothers' lives, can be practiced directly in the context for which they are meant.

At times, treatment of trauma survivors is not appropriate for the telehealth format if the client is dysregulated by the lack of direct coregulation that face-to-face treatment offers. Lack of privacy can also be an issue. It is important to explain the ongoing assessment of the appropriateness of telehealth to the client from the beginning of treatment, as part of the informed consent, and carefully consider the client's options. If the alternative to telehealth treatment is no treatment at all, the therapist can consider adjusting the treatment goal to focus on attunement, stabilizing, and psychoeducation, and avoid deeper processing of traumatic themes until the client has either developed a greater capacity to regulate or can get access to in-person treatment. In this situation, the therapist must be diligent with appropriate referrals and resources that support the client outside of therapy sessions (this will be elaborated in Chapter 8).

Clinician Self-Reflection

The ideological layers of the cultural expectations of motherhood are constantly present in our work with mothers, especially in the somatic transferential field of perinatal therapy. Therapists must acknowledge this in their ongoing self-scrutiny and processing of their countertransference reactions. We all carry projections onto the maternal body, the maternal subject, the mother-infant couple, the realm of the perinatal transition and its bodily relations, and the mothering practices that are non-conforming relative to the dictates of patriarchal or normative motherhood. The attuned perinatal therapist has dedicated themselves to continuously build awareness of their personal maternally themed projections and how these projections relate to their own trauma history. The following self-reflection questions are meant for perinatal therapists to deepen their awareness of the maternal themes in their somatic countertransference reactions, ideally in the context of supervision, consultation, or personal therapy:

- What type of mothering practices can activate your judgment?
- What types of mothering situations do you find the most stressful to witness?
- What mothering situations do you associate with shame?
- How do you respond to being in the presence of newborns and infants? And the new mother?
- What somatic reactions do you most often have when being in the presence of new mothers and babies?
- What are your experiences of this from both your professional and personal life?
- What mothering or parenting philosophy do you resonate with the most?
- What body states, narratives, and values related to the maternal body are prevalent in that philosophy?

- What mothering or parenting philosophy do you resonate with the least and feel the most negative feelings about? Why?
- What motherhood ideology or philosophy have you had the strongest reactions to?
- How much of these reactions are related to your own experience of mothering or not mothering?
- What is your relationship with maternal bodies? Your own, your own mother's, other family members or friends who are mothers, other non-mothers fulfilling maternal or caregiving roles?
- What happens in your body when you listen to stories related to maternal body transitions and mothering?
- Which maternal body themes do you find most activating or challenging to listen to? What do you know about your own history, including your trauma history, that could relate to this?
- What are the aspects of embodied mothering you find the most challenging to process somatically?
- Which bodily aspects of mothering do you find yourself feeling neutral or positive towards?

References

Ackerman, M., Greenwald, E., Noulas, P., & Ahn, C. (2021). Patient satisfaction with and use of telemental health services in the perinatal period: A survey study. *Psychiatric Quarterly*, *92*(3), 925–933. 10.1007/s11126-020-09874-8

Beebe, B., & Lachmann, F. (1988). The contribution of mother-infant mutual influence to the origins of self- and object representations. *Psychoanalytic Psychology*, *5*, 305–337. 10.1037/0736-9735.5.4.305

Caldwell, C.M. (2016) Body identity development: Definitions and discussions. *Body, Movement and Dance in Psychotherapy*, *11*(4), 220–234. 10.1080/17432979.2016.1145141

Caldwell, C.M. (2018a). *Bodyfulness. Somatic practices for presence, empowerment, and waking up in this life*. Shambala.

Caldwell, C.M. (2018b). Body identity development: Who we are and who we become. In C.M. Caldwell, & L.B. Leighton (Eds.), *Oppression and the body. Roots, resistance, and resolutions* (pp. 31–50). North Atlantic Books.

Carroll, R. (2014). Four relational modes of attending to the body. In K. White (Ed.), *Talking bodies. How do we integrate working with the body in psychotherapy from an attachment and relational perspective. The John Bowlby Memorial Conference Monograph 2012* (pp. 11–39). Routledge. 10.4324/9780429480812

Harrang, C., Tillotson, D., & Winters, N.C. (2022). General introduction. In C. Harrang, D. Tillotson, & N.C. Winters (Eds.), *Body as psychoanalytic object. Clinical applications from Winnicott to Bion and beyond* (pp. 1–9). Routledge. 10.4324/9781003195559

Hill, D. (2015). *Affect regulation theory. A clinical model.* Norton.

Johnson, K.A. (2021). *Call of the wild: How we heal trauma, awaken our own power, and use it for good.* Harper Wave.

Kuhfuß, M., Maldei, T., Hetmanek, A., & Baumann, N. (2021). Somatic experiencing – effectiveness and key factors of a body-oriented trauma therapy: A scoping literature review. *European Journal of Psychotraumatology, 12*, 1929023. 10.1080/20008198.2021.1929023

Kumar, N.R., Arias, M.P., Leitner, K., Wang, E., Clement, E.G., & Hamm, R.F. (2022). Assessing the impact of telehealth implementation on postpartum outcomes for Black birthing people. *American Journal of Obstetrics & Gynecology MFM, 5*(2), 100831. Advance online publication. 10.1016/j.ajogmf.2022.100831

LaPierre, A. (2015). Relational body psychotherapy (or relational somatic psychology). *International Body Psychotherapy Journal, 14*(2), 80–100.

Leddick, K.H. (2018). Making good use of combined therapeutic modalities: Discussion of "Somatic Experiencing". *Psychoanalytic Dialogues, 28*(5), 610–619. 10.1080/10481885.2018.1506223

Levine, P.A. (2010). *In an unspoken voice. How the body releases trauma and restores goodness.* North Atlantic Books.

Levine, P.A., Blakeslee, A., & Sylvae, J. (2018). Reintegrating fragmentation of the primitive self: Discussion of "Somatic Experiencing", *Psychoanalytic Dialogues, 28*(5), 620–628, 10.1080/10481885.2018.1506216

Orbach, S. (2006). How can we have a body?: Desires and corporeality. *Studies In Gender & Sexuality*, *7*(1), 89–111.

Orbach, S. (2009). *Bodies*. Picador.

Payne, P., Levine, P.A., & Crane-Godreau, M.A. (2015). Somatic experiencing: Using interoception and proprioception as core elements of trauma therapy. *Frontiers in Psychology*, *6*, 93. 10.3389/fpsyg.2015.00093

Polmanteer, R.S.R., Keefe, R.H., & Brownstein-Evans, C. (2019). Trauma-informed care with women diagnosed with postpartum depression: A conceptual framework. *Social Work in Health Care*, *58*(2), 220–235. 10.1080/00981389.2018.1535464

Porges, S.W. (2022). Polyvagal theory: A science of safety. *Frontiers in Integrative Neuroscience*, *16*, 871227. 10.3389/fnint.2022.871227

Schore, A.N. (1998). Early shame experiences and infant brain development. In P. Gilbert, & B. Andrews (Eds.), *Shame: Interpersonal behavior, psychopathology, and culture* (pp. 57–77). Oxford University Press.

Schore, A.N. (2012). *The science of the art of psychotherapy*. Norton.

Schore, A.N. (2021). The interpersonal neurobiology of intersubjectivity. *Frontiers in Psychology*, *12*, 648616. 10.3389/fpsyg.2021.648616

Selvam, R. (2022). *The practice of embodying emotions. A guide for improving cognitive, emotional, and behavioral outcomes*. North Atlantic Books.

Wassef, A., & Wassef, E. (2022). Telemedicine in perinatal mental health: Perspectives. *Journal of Psychosomatic Obstetrics and Gynecology*, *43*(2), 224–227. 10.1080/0167482X.2021.2024162

Zhao, L., Chen, J., Lan, L., Deng, N., Liao, Y., Yue, L., Chen, I., Wen, S.W., & Xie, R.H. (2021). Effectiveness of telehealth interventions for women with postpartum depression: Systematic review and meta-analysis. *JMIR mHealth and uHealth*, *9*(10), e32544. 10.2196/32544

6

Maternal Bodyfulness
Working with Perinatal Sensory Awareness and Vocabulary

Emotion Regulation and Sensory Awareness in the Perinatal Period

Emotion regulation involves a coherent relationship with oneself, including communication between body, mind, and feelings (Price & Hooven, 2018), and is acknowledged to influence us deeply, possibly every aspect of our functioning (Rutherford et al., 2015). Research has demonstrated that effective emotion regulation depends on the ability to detect and evaluate interoceptive cues related to physiological reactions and use that information to strategize a response, further corroborated by a significant amount of evidence demonstrating links between poor sensory awareness and emotional regulation difficulties (Price & Hooven, 2018). Emotion regulatory function during the perinatal period is recognized as distinct from emotion regulation during other periods of life (Rutherford et al., 2015). The perinatal period is a time of increasing and new forms of sensations, unlike any other life stage. Perinatal sensations cover a wide range of sensations that are often contrasting, for example, the pleasure of touching and smelling one's newborn while simultaneously feeling the muscle pain from childbirth recovery. The perinatal period is unique because the mother has to maintain a regulated state herself while also facilitating regulation in her child, posing a significant challenge to her emotion regulation system (Rutherford et al., 2015). The sensory aspects of the maternal transition are especially challenging for the first-time mother who doesn't have a reference to make sense of them. It is no surprise that emotion regulation is challenging for the new mother. Subsequent pregnancies and postpartum transitions are unique and bring new bodily experiences different from the first. The perinatal period involves an overwhelming number of new sensations occurring while the new mother is undergoing a recalibration of her entire sensory and regulatory system.

Perinatal sensations are not limited to the discomforts of childbirth recovery but play a central role in the development of the coregulatory relationship between mother and infant. The new perinatal sensations interweave with feelings, meanings, memories, relational interactions, and emotion regulation dynamics, producing a concoction of experiences that fertilize the developing maternal sense of self and fuel bonding and coregulation. As the nervous system moves into a profoundly coregulating mode in the perinatal period, the sensory processing activity is increased, and emotion regulation dynamics are reorganized. New neuroscience studies suggest that brain changes associated with the mother's physiological reaction to infant cues postpartum are occurring already during pregnancy (Hoekzema et al., 2022). Effective attunement to and coregulation with a newborn requires a capacity to use interoceptive, exteroceptive, and proprioceptive experiential knowledge for intersubjective relating. The therapeutic relationship must also adapt to this mode of "shared psychosensory experience" (Harrang et al., 2022). The work of mothering is widely acknowledged as emotionally challenging, but a mother's work of adjusting and adapting her sensory processing capacities for the purpose of regulating herself and her baby is rarely fully appreciated, let alone verbally acknowledged. Working actively with sensory awareness in perinatal therapy will unfold a comprehensive layer of coregulation experiences that connects to the new mother's developing embodied subjectivity as well as her trauma history.

Sensory awareness is central to bottom-up trauma treatment and a cornerstone of self-regulation (Levine, 2010). It is by definition experiential, a phenomenon of experience, not just a characteristic of perception. It is more than awareness of sensations; it is about building a relationship with and a full experience of sensation (Caldwell, 2018a). Furthermore, it is about the ability to make use of this sensory information for emotion regulation. Sensory awareness is both the foundation and the result of self-regulation, an infinite loop of interactions. The more regulated we are, the more aware we are of our sensations and vice versa. To be well-regulated is to be able to make good use of sensations as opposed to either ignoring or actively numbing them (Levine, 2010). This requires us to slow down. Slowing down is necessary for effective tracking of our sensations. This is paralleled by the necessity to slow down our mental activity to identify and process our thoughts and emotions. Feeling rushed is in direct opposition to being regulated. Slowing down enables us to make better use of our sensations as information for self-regulation. For many, slowing down will in and of itself increase regulation. For others, slowing down might be experienced as activating and frustrating because they are habituated to rushing as a way to cope with sensations that are hard to tolerate, or because slowing down is associated with a lack of safety due to traumatic imprints of chronic autonomic over-activation.

Slowing down in service of regulation can feel like an unattainable luxury for the new mother who is constantly attending to the needs of her baby. Mothering has a paradoxical quality of simultaneously feeling slowed down due to daily life being primarily formed around the needs and rhythms of the baby and feeling accelerated due to the baby's needs being immediate, constant, and largely unpredictable. Pausing to attend to sensations can seem counterintuitive when mothering. Mothering involves adaptive impulses to actively anticipate and predict the baby's needs, which increases nervous system activation. The inherent physiological stressors of the perinatal period make it challenging to slow down. This is further pronounced by traumatic stress, both in the case of pre-existing chronic patterns of autonomic dysregulation and in the case of recent acute trauma. Expectations and goals for the perinatal client's ability to slow down must be realistic and sensitive to the realities of mothering as well as thoroughly informed by the client's trauma history. However, it must not be given up, no matter how unrealistic it might seem like for the overwhelmed client. Even the smallest amounts of progress with practicing slowing down are valuable in the treatment process.

Being regulated by using sensations effectively must also be experienced as a choice, an act of agency. According to Levine (2010), sensations are the bedrock of autonomy and independence. Although our regulation capacities are formed from coregulation, regulation must ultimately become self-directed in the context of trauma healing. It is the experience of agency in one's sensory awareness that counters the feeling states of powerlessness that characterize trauma and makes sensations tolerable to work with and through. When we have agency in our felt sense, we can experience our sensations as waves we can ride, as opposed to waves that come thrashing over us. The experience of agency in navigating sensations undergoes a reorganization in the perinatal transition where new sensations and nervous system dynamics, including those of the baby, must be integrated. It is a steep learning curve to develop agency in the navigation of new perinatal sensations, often eliciting frustrations. Sensory awareness skills help to regulate the new mother as she is reworking her relationship with her new maternal body and its unique sensations and her coregulation relationship with her baby. Regulation relates to both increasing her felt sense of bodily experiences in the context of limited connection to positive and stabilizing sensations and lowering the intensity of sensations in the context of overwhelm. While some clients have a tendency for one of these, many experience shifting between them depending on context. The tendency to numb or ignore sensations to reduce experiences of negative sensations comes with the high price of reducing experiences of positive sensations. The underlying issue for both tendencies is a lack of somatic agency: The ability to influence the intensity level of sensation by actively shifting attention, down- or upregulating stimulation, and responding effectively to interoceptive and proprioceptive information. Somatic agency is necessary for building affect tolerance. Sensory awareness skills both reduce internal overwhelm and build tolerance for it, thereby supporting the processing of affects. The more regulatory access a person has to their entire range of bodily sensations, the better they are able to process intense affects (Selvam, 2022). The wide range of affects that characterizes the maternal transition calls for the expansion of the capacity to tolerate sensations.

In the therapeutic situation, sensory awareness is more than awareness of sensations. To make therapeutic use of sensations, they must be tracked in real-time by the therapeutic couple, so the client has a coregulatory experience of being witnessed in the present moment. Sensory awareness skills begin with the therapist's tracking of their own and the client's nervous system, as described in Chapter 5. Most clients and therapists without somatic training are unfamiliar with this, and for some, it can feel awkward. To effectively track sensations, it is necessary to slow down the pace of the entire relational interaction and the person's inner state. For clients with high levels of traumatic stress, this can be very challenging, especially if they don't feel relationally safe. Sensory awareness is a practical skill, but it is instigated in the client through the attuned coregulatory therapeutic relationship. We cannot teach a client to track their sensations without doing this ourselves simultaneously and offering our witnessing of the client's experience of sensations. The primary somatic listening skills of tracking one's own and the client's nervous system are intertwined. In other words, the attuned therapist listens to the body and responds accordingly, parallel to the mother's constant coregulation with her baby.

When clients struggle with the unfamiliar experience of intentionally tracking their sensations in real-time in the therapeutic situation, the therapist must be careful to acknowledge and attune to this discomfort and dysregulation to normalize that sensory awareness practice is difficult, especially in the perinatal period where sensory processing systems are undergoing significant changes. A key principle for reducing overwhelm is to shift attention to exteroceptive experiences (experiencing the environment) when interoception (internal sensations) feels overwhelming (Johnson, 2021). When the client is supported in shifting back and forth between exteroception and interoception tracking at their own pace and noticing their immediate responses, they are developing somatic agency. The demands of caring for a baby can easily override a mother's feelings of agency in her self-regulation, even more so for the mother who already struggled with somatic agency before becoming a mother. The constant tracking of the baby's cues can make an anxious mother feel powerless, understandably so. Some mothers become intensively focused on tracking their babies at the expense of their own sensory awareness, especially if they had prior tendencies for hypervigilant tracking of others as a result of developmental trauma. The coregulation of the therapeutic situation facilitates reciprocal and intersubjective awareness where both the client's and the therapist's states are valued in the co-creation of the interaction.

The therapeutic situation of slowing down, engaging the client in real-time tracking of their sensations, and supporting their sense of somatic agency must be done with an attitude of non-judgmental curiosity (see Figure 6.1 for an overview of the foundations of sensory awareness). In general, new mothers are often highly sensitive to feeling judged and struggle with internal self-judgment, and this is pronounced for mothers who are depressed, anxious, or traumatized. Experiencing a lack of safety in a relational interaction impacts the way and the degree to which a person engages in coregulation (Porges, 2022) and their sense of agency (Hill, 2015). A non-judgmental attitude is crucial when working clinically with sensory awareness to ensure the therapeutic safety that is a prerequisite for effective coregulation. This attitude is communicated both verbally via invitational language and psychoeducation and nonverbally via the therapist's embodied uninhibited openness to the client's experiences. The non-judgmental attitude is also crucial for supporting a new mother's assertion of her own way of mothering, in opposition to dictates of normative motherhood and parenting ideologies.

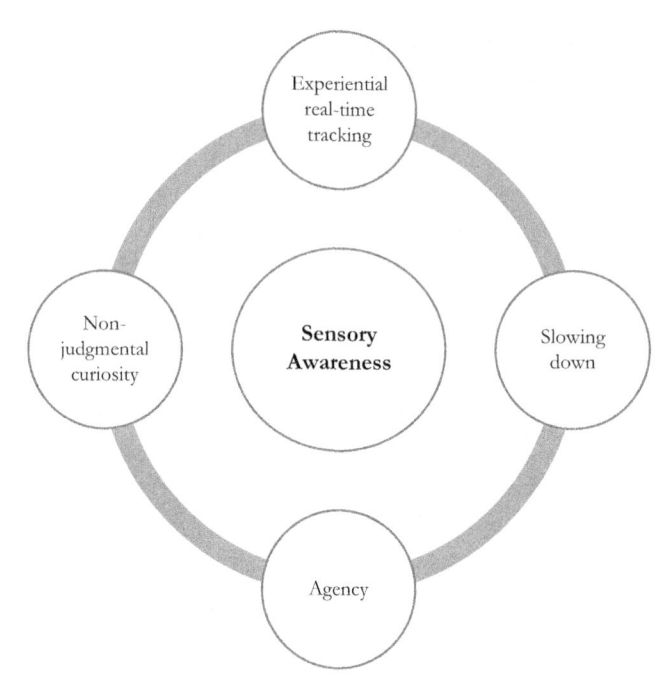

FIGURE 6.1 Foundations of Sensory Awareness

Maternal Sense of Self, Sensory Awareness, and Pleasure

Levine (2010) contends that sensory awareness is central to the sense of self and therefore concludes that loss of sensations leads to a loss of sense of self. Self-regulation patterns are unique reflections of an individual's sense of self and developmental history. To work on sensory awareness is to indirectly work on the bodily sense of self. Body narratives and body identity development are relationally formed and experienced (Caldwell, 2016; LaPierre, 2015), as is the new mother's emerging maternal body identity. As identity is transformed by becoming a mother, the bodily sense of self and thereby self-regulation is also shifted. The maternal transition involves not only a revisiting, but a reworking of the body narrative and body identity history, especially its self-regulation aspects. The maternal subject position cannot be conceived only on a mental level; it is conferred by the somatic experience of becoming a maternal body. Working on the level of sensory awareness concretizes and captures the experiential foundation of the abstract notion of identity transformation. If we wish to support the new mother in processing her feelings of loss of self, it is not enough to present the abstract idea of her sense of self as the antidote. Sensations are the strata of the body narrative that evolves into an embodied sense of self (Caldwell, 2018b). Working with sensory awareness, therefore, offers more granularity for the new sense of maternal self. Sensory awareness is central to maternal bodyfulness, as it is about building trust in sensations as possible healing agents. Maternal bodyfulness is the appreciation of sensations as fuel for an embodied sense of self and, by extension, perinatal sensations as foundational to the maternal sense of self. Here, perinatal sensations are not seen as obstacles to be overcome or polished into positive forms, but as the underpinnings of the experience of coming into one's maternal subjectivity.

Pleasure plays a crucial role in the development of maternal subjectivity and maternal bodyfulness. Sensory experiences of pleasure have a central function in the developing relationship with the baby (Piccini, 2021), where the coregulatory patterns of interaction between mother and child are dependent on the mother's neurological reward system (Strathearn et al., 2008; Schore, 2021). But pleasure must also be considered from the mother's perspective alone. The ability to stay present to pleasurable sensations is stabilizing (Johnson, 2021). The new mother is in dire need of stabilization as she undergoes the destabilization of the maternal transition. As discussed in Chapter 1, the assumption in Western culture that maternal subjectivity is in opposition to the individual challenges our recognition of mothers as full subjects. De Marneffe (2004) has pointed out that when we internalize the discourses of motherhood being antithetical to self, it profoundly impacts our ability to recognize and experience maternal desires and maternal gratification as positive aspects of self. Mothers can struggle with acknowledging the positive and pleasurable aspects of mothering as part of their struggle to be recognized and recognize themselves as full subjects, especially in the culture of intensive mothering ideology that dictates that mothering should be primarily demanding and focused on self-sacrifice. Valuing pleasure and positive sensations requires an underlying assumption of them as important to one's subject position as well as a sense of being deserving of them.

As sensations form the bodily sense of self, a mother's positive sense of self relies on positive sensory experiences of maternal embodiment and mothering. A mother's somatic receptivity (her relationship with the felt experience of receiving, see Chapter 5) is formed by experiences of sensory pleasure from receiving. Barriers to mothers experiencing the pleasurable aspects of mothering fully can be related to the individual and cultural stigma around somatic receptivity. If mothers are empowered in their experience of the pleasurable aspects of mothering, they are resisting the dictates of normative motherhood and intensive mothering ideology that stipulate that mothers must always put their children's needs before their own and that mothering is meant to be intense. Claiming pleasure in the context of mothering can therefore be understood as a form of resistance against patriarchal motherhood, an empowered mothering practice. However, the capacity to feel pleasurable sensations depends on general sensory awareness and tolerance of all forms of sensations. Experiential knowledge of pleasant sensations is also necessary for trauma healing because it contradicts the sensations of traumatic overwhelm and thus facilitates neurological habituation of the experience of being regulated (Johnson, 2021; Levine et al., 2018). Through the practicing of awareness of positive sensations, the body is discovered as a resource in itself, a cornerstone of somatic trauma healing (Kuhfuß et al., 2021), and one's experiential capacity is expanded (Johnson, 2021).

The Impact of Perinatal Trauma on Sensory Awareness and the Therapeutic Relationship

The sensations of pregnancy, delivery, and postpartum can be very distressing and activating for trauma survivors, especially in cases with a history of childhood or adult sexual abuse and traumatic childbirth (Granner & Seng, 2021; Simkin & Klaus, 2004).

Perinatal sensations can activate dissociated traumatic body memories which may or may not be available for conscious processing. Even though positive, sensual, or pleasurable sensations in the perinatal period are central to both mother-infant bonding and the mother's development of an embodied sense of maternal self, they can also be experienced as unsafe or activating traumatic body memories. This is because positive sensations have been associated with traumatic memories. Dysregulation comes in different degrees of intensity and scope, but it always challenges our sensory awareness. It either sends us away from being connected to our sensations or causes us to be consumed by them, in temporary bursts or for prolonged periods of time. Dysregulation is generally understood as prolonged activation of the nervous system, from increased heart rate to our fight and flight impulses, and a lack of release or completion of the responses that are necessary for down-regulating and resettling. Both pre-existing trauma and trauma that occurred in the perinatal transition can therefore interfere with the mother's ability to stay connected to her sensations. The new maternal role entails protecting both baby and self in their shared vulnerability, which will activate psychobiological systems of survival, including aggression. When survival systems are overloaded from trauma, toxic stress, or allostatic load, anger, and rage reaction patterns can become chronically over-active. A common defense against affective overwhelm is splitting off, causing a disconnect from experiences of pleasure. Lack of pleasure and joy in the perinatal period related to affective overwhelm and traumatic stress is deeply problematic not only because of the immediate depressogenic effect, but also because of its insidious inhibition of the mother's development of embodied maternal subjectivity.

Sensory awareness brings up more than sensations. It brings up emotions, cognitions, meanings, narratives, images, and memories. In the case of childhood maltreatment and attachment trauma, the new mother might have internalized negative associations related to all sensations, or a state of being generally averse to sensations. A somatic consequence of insecure attachment is a negative or rigid relationship to sensations where regulation can be experienced as a power struggle with the body. As discussed in Chapter 1, the trauma of insecure attachment is entrenched in the bodily sense of self which becomes insecure. This body insecurity (Orbach, 2009) or bodylessness (Caldwell, 2018a) manifests in a person's relationship to sensations. Although the maternal transition can magnify body insecurity, it can also be an opportunity to rework one's entire relationship with sensations. However, being asked to engage with sensations can easily be experienced as intolerable by trauma survivors. The therapist must offer a reframing of the associations of sensations as something negative and related to rupture, abandonment, and frustration to an experience of agency, where the client chooses to attend to sensations to make use of them for self-regulation. This reframing can be offered explicitly with words but is primarily communicated through the therapist's nonverbal coregulatory somatic attunement and embodied attitude towards the client's body and self-regulation capacities.

The sensory experiences of both the maternal transition and trauma range from fragmented, incoherent, elusive, confusing, and even volatile at times. It is crucial that clinicians can work non-judgmentally with this range. For clients with a nervous system history of a preponderance of overwhelm, the normal cycles of activation and deactivation have been interrupted, reflected in dysregulation patterns that impact the sense of self and beliefs about one's body and self-regulation capacities. It is important to adopt a stance of accepting the client's negative feelings towards their body sensations. Clinicians must not deny the client's experience of body hatred and resistance to tracking sensations, but instead cultivate curiosity about it (Orbach, 2006). The new mother's negative feelings about her maternal body and sensations must be explored in the context of her altered subjectivity, her ambivalence, and her developmental history to understand the underlying components of trauma. The experience of mothering becomes less rewarding when a mother has unresolved trauma (Iyengar et al., 2019). The survival responses related to trauma impact the mother's sensory awareness through the over-activation of the autonomous nervous system activation. This makes it harder for her to build new experiential knowledge of the positive rewarding sensations of mothering which are crucial for her adjustment and enjoyment of the coregulatory interactions with her baby. The absence of any sensory awareness of pleasure, joy, and gratification in a new mother's reports of her daily life should prompt clinical attention and exploration.

Sensory awareness is central to the trauma-healing process because it is through our physical body sensations we can access and work with the instinctual survival responses that are interrupted by trauma (Levine, 2010). In my clinical experience, some mothers with severe developmental trauma have never experienced a caregiving relationship in which the other had a conscious and intentional positive attitude towards their body and self-regulation capacities. Some clients describe not having experienced any feelings or thoughts at all from their caregivers about their capacities for sensation and regulation. In some cases, this made the client fill in a sense of meaning in the absence of it, with that meaning often reflecting their state of despair or shame about not being recognized by their caregiver in a coregulatory sense. For those clients, working with sensory awareness can seem threatening, foreign, even outlandish. The bodily developmental history is at the center here. A caregiver's perception of a child's bodily capacities deeply influences the child's development of their relationship with their body (Orbach, 2011). The new mother with insecure attachment is undergoing a reactivation of the early developmental history of her relationship with her body stemming from her relationship with her own mother and caregivers. Working with sensory awareness is directed at the client's relationship to her body: The therapist must offer the client an experience of being met with a positive attitude towards her body and her capacities for self-regulation. The therapist's attitude towards the client's body and body capacities is connected to the therapist's attitude towards their own body and regulation capacities, making it important for therapists to maintain attentiveness to somatic countertransference and personal patterns of somatic bias reactions (see Chapter 5).

Introducing Sensory Awareness Skills to Perinatal Clients

Sensory awareness skills build on the clinical tools of attunement, resonance, and nervous system tracking presented in Chapter 5. Working with sensory awareness skills comes into focus when the perinatal therapist has 1. established therapeutic coregulatory safety using resonance, 2. actively tracked and sat with the client's dysregulation, and 3. cultivated and addressed barriers to somatic receptivity (see Chapter 5). A basic way to introduce sensory awareness is to introduce the topics of bodily stability, pleasure, and gratification in mothering. The following reflection questions are meant to build awareness, curiosity, and vocabulary about the sensory aspects of mothering. They can be revisited and should not be seen as a one-time exercise to be completed.

Sensory Awareness Reflection Questions

- When do you feel the best or the most stable in your body?
- When do you feel the most joy when caring for your baby? When do you feel the most calm or stable?
- What are the most pleasurable parts of caring for your baby? What kinds of activities or times of the day?
- What places, surroundings, or activities can make caring for your baby feel good or better in your body?
- How does it feel in your body right when your baby stops crying or settles? What does that moment feel like in your body, when things calm down?

For clients with high levels of distress who report having little to no positive sensations, the parameters should be adjusted to ask about neutral sensations. Questions can also be framed to differentiate degrees of negative sensations, e.g., "When do you feel the least tense in your body? What parts of caring for your baby feel the least stressful?" This reframing can be necessary when working with clients with high levels of stress who have primarily negative associations with sensations, especially when establishing therapeutic safety. It is also an opportunity to sit with and attune to the client's dysregulation and offer empathy when the client reports not having any positive or pleasurable sensations. However, it is also important to psychoeducate clients in a timely and sensitive way about the link between emotion regulation and sensory awareness and that healing trauma will eventually involve developing a more positive relationship with sensations through sensory awareness practice. The aim of such psychoeducation is to convey hope and communicate confidence in the client's capacities for improving their regulation with practice (see the section on psychoeducation in Chapter 8). Therapists must be careful to avoid putting pressure on the client by calling into focus the principle of non-judgmental curiosity. A helpful message here is that everyone has the capacity for developing self-regulating sensory awareness skills as they are founded on our innate mammalian psychobiology. This message relocates the client's bodily experiential knowledge as the authority.

Somatic Self-Regulation Skills

Sensory awareness is the cornerstone of self-regulation. When interoceptive awareness is developed, sensory information can be used effectively to modify one's internal state. It is not enough to only pay attention to high-intensity sensations that stand out and are impossible to ignore. For effective self-regulation, it is important to develop ongoing awareness of all sensations and their continuing changes, including neutral and low-intensity sensations. When the threshold of sensory awareness is lowered, the range of sensations experienced is widened, so low-intensity sensations are incorporated into self-regulation strategies. Self-regulation requires ongoing tracking of both sensory and experiential shifts in nervous system activation and the new experiences that emerge in response to one's self-regulatory movements and behaviors. The somatic agency of initiating and halting behaviors to self-regulate relies on experiential knowledge of one's body and openness to registering new sensations and reactions. The combined use of tracking and intentionally changing one's inner state is then directed at connecting to a felt sense of relative safety in the here and now. Somatic self-regulation does not depend on the ability to verbalize all aspects of sensory awareness. A large amount of self-regulation happens outside of verbalization. However, language can be conducive to sensory awareness building, but it requires an approach to cultivating sensory vocabulary. See Table 6.1 for an overview of somatic self-regulation skills and Appendix B for a description of exercises for each skill.

TABLE 6.1 Somatic Self-Regulation Skills

Somatic Self-Regulation Skills

Felt sense, sensory awareness	Ongoing sensory awareness of internal state and ability to identify and distinguish between different sensations.
External awareness	Experiential awareness of immediate surroundings with all senses.
Grounding	Sensing gravity to create a felt sense of stability and connection.
Checking of activation levels	Noticing and tracking changes in nervous system activation levels.
Up- and down-regulating	Using internal and external awareness shifts to down- or up-regulate stimulation.
Monitoring	Tracking the effects of attention-shifting on internal state.
Regulating movements	Intentional and paced use of movements, posture shifts, or self-touch to modify internal state.
Slowing down (healthy inhibition)	Ability to halt, slow down, or modify movements, postures, and states that are contributing to dysregulation.
Somatic agency	Ability to identify and follow impulses to make regulating movements.
Establish relative safety	Using all of the above to establish and confirm the experience of relative safety in the here-and-now.

Sensory Vocabulary and Maternal Body Narrative

Mothering makes it challenging to achieve coherence in one's body narrative. The constant interruptions of motherwork make it hard to experience a flow in one's going on being of daily life (Baraitser, 2009). Furthermore, our language does not adequately cover the unique sensory aspects of mothering. Phillips (2022) has noted that many parental sensations don't have words. Caldwell (2018a) reminds us that our language is limited when it comes to bodily experiences and only offers approximations of them. For the maternal transition, this is even more pronounced by the erasure of maternal embodied subjectivity. We have only recently begun to see conversations in the public realm and media discourses about the sensory experiences of pregnancy, delivery, and postpartum, and these conversations often address the inherent taboo, stigma, and lack of acknowledgment and language about perinatal experiences. Speaking to the sensations and the bodily experience of the perinatal period is even seen as an act of rebellion, defiance, resistance, or something radical. The sensations and bodily aspects of the maternal transition are communicated against the backdrop of the silencing of maternal subjectivity. In the same way, the bodily experience of trauma has a limited place in daily language. The new mother with trauma has precious little exposure to sensory vocabulary that captures her experience.

Building sensory vocabulary with the perinatal client is a work of discovering and creating personalized language. The goal of such language building is not to verbalize all aspects of a mother's maternal body narrative and identity, but to support her perinatal sensory awareness and her agency and authority in her conscious discovery and experience of her embodied sense of her maternal self. We must avoid any pressure to develop vocabulary with the purpose of making coherent, logical, and explanatory narratives. Sensory vocabulary is primarily about supporting sensory awareness and is often incoherent, guttural, and fragmented (Johnson, 2021). The meaning-making and coherence that can evolve from such vocabulary are maximized when the body's rhythms are made present in speech. Sensory vocabulary are the words that help the client deepen their felt sense or capture a feeling state and thereby help the client integrate and attend to it. Maternal sensory vocabulary is a way to bring language back to the maternal body, thereby both acknowledging and inviting the unconscious visceral realm of the maternal transition, expanding the possibilities for integration of it. This interplay between verbal and nonverbal levels of processing nurtures the synergistic relationship between body narratives and explicit self-narratives and facilitates the integration of unconscious material.

As discussed in Chapter 5, the perinatal therapist must adopt a mindset of prioritizing somatic attunement over cognitive understanding to ensure therapeutic safety. This is important when cultivating sensory vocabulary to avoid putting pressure on the client to produce verbal coherence and intellectual meaning. Effective emotional regulation requires hemispheric integration, meaning left-brain-dominated language-based cognitions must be connected with right-brain-dominated felt affects (Hill, 2015). The purpose of verbalizing the sensory experience of the maternal transition is to support regulation capacities by facilitating hemispheric integration. Sensory vocabulary is meant to support the developing maternal body narrative that is the foundation of maternal embodied subjectivity. When Beck (2017) investigated the language used by women with birth-related PTSD, she discovered that they used metaphorical expressions to capture the intensity of their traumatic experiences. Maternal sensory vocabulary is different from emotional and intellectual language. It will often be metaphorical and symbolic or include idiosyncratic references, associations, and expressions. It might have elements of motherese, prosodic playfulness, or onomatopoeia. From my clinical experience, mothers often rely on wordplays and humorous expressions, especially with sarcasm or irony, to capture their embodied experiences of the maternal transition. Parker (1995) concluded from her qualitative research with mothers that maternal ambivalence, which is notoriously hard for mothers to talk about due to shame and stigma, is often tolerated better through the use of humor, if it is talked about at all. Whether a mother uses humorous remarks or doesn't have any words for her bodily experiences, the therapist must sensitively invite collaborative exploration of her vocabulary related to sensations and bodily topics.

Table 6.2 is a non-exhaustive list of sensory words organized by the categories of intensity, movement and direction, skin, temperature, constriction, and expansion. The list does not indicate that sensory vocabulary should be rigidly organized but is meant solely as a starting point for exploration, especially for clients who have limited sensory vocabulary, to begin with. Several words may double in more than one category. The list can be used for the therapist's reference and practice of attuning to sensory vocabulary in sessions, or it can be shared with the client as a psychoeducational resource depending on the client's needs and preferences.

Maternal Bodyfulness Themes in Trauma Healing

Trauma healing has long been understood as a process of naming and speaking the truth of one's experience as a way to break the silence and reclaim agency, connecting the act of verbalizing to empowerment. For example, in Bernard and Bernard's (1998) definition of empowerment: "Empowerment is naming, analyzing, and challenging oppression on an individual, collective, and/or structural level" (p. 46). However, verbal language is limited for perinatal trauma processing for several reasons. As mentioned, cultural vocabulary about perinatal sensations is limited. Furthermore, as perinatal sensations can activate traumatic memories, even talking about them can cause activation in some clients. They may not always realize why they have arousal responses to seemingly neutral conversation topics common in the perinatal context. Mothers who experience hyperarousal from unconscious trauma reactions may experience confusion or shame about their reactions which is easily exacerbated by insensitive or judgmental surroundings.

Somatic trauma processing does not require the client to be able to work with clear and coherent narratives and explanations of objective facts. In fact, it is conducive to suspend any

TABLE 6.2 Sensation Words

Intensity	Movement & direction	Skin	Temperature	Constriction	Expansion
Calm	Bubbly	Clammy	Blazing	Blocked	Bloating
Consistent	Building	Cracked	Boiling	Bound	Building
Dull	Collapsing	Dry	Burning	Clasped	Discharging
Evenly	Dripping	Electric	Chill	Clenched	Drooping
Explosive	Dripping	Flushing	Cold	Closed	Energized
Forceful	Drooping	Irritable	Cool	Collapsed	Expanding
Hard	Dwindling	Itchy	Cooling	Compressed	Explosive
Heavy	Expanding	Moist	Firey	Confined	Filling
Indistinct	Exploding	Numb	Frozen	Congested	Floaty
Intense	Falling	Oily	Hot	Contracted	Flowing
Light	Fizzling out	Prickly	Icy	Cut-off	Fluid
Loose	Flowing	Quivery	Luke-warm	Knotted	Freeing
Neutral	Imploding	Soggy	Room temperature	Pressured	Glowing
Piercing	Lifting	Sore	Scalding	Pulled	Growing
Pounding	Moving	Stinging	Scorching	Pushed	Loosening
Pressured	Pulsating	Sweaty	Steamy	Solid	Opening
Sharp	Shrinking	Tender	Tepid	Stuck	Radiating
Soft	Sinking	Tingling	Thawing	Sucked	Releasing
Still	Slowing	Touchy	Toasty	Tense	Releasing
Subtle	Streaming Waving	Trembling	Warm	Tethered	Spacious
Vague	Wobbly	Twitchy	White-hot	Tight	Stretching
Weak		Wet		Weighted	Vibrating

expectations for verbal neatness and coherence and tune into how the rhythms of sensations manifest through language. The verbal language used in sessions does not account for all of the treatment happening, nor should the therapist attempt to verbalize everything that is happening. The core of somatic therapy is the sensory experiences happening in the coregulation field. Levine et al. (2018) describe how working with the body narrative by attending to the somatic cues before interpreting the verbal narrative is important when integrating unconscious material to support a return to the embodied sense of self. As Johnson (2021) has pointed out, "we can't think or talk our way toward healing" (p. xix).

The language of the body is helpful when capturing and processing the upheaval of the maternal transition and the way this upheaval is pronounced by trauma, but only if the language is used in a way that supports sensory awareness and coregulation. The somatically attuned therapist maintains a level of curiosity about the client's sensory experience of verbalizing that is not exceeded by their curiosity about the factual content of the trauma narrative. At times it is necessary to suspend any verbalizing of the trauma story to help the client orient to the present moment through sensory awareness, to prevent or resolve overwhelm (Levine, 2010). Signs of overwhelm from verbalizing traumatic memories are characterized by symptoms of dysregulation including blunt or flat expression of affect, pressured or slowed down speech, hyperventilating, monotony, intense emotionality, and lack of coherence. The lack of a coherent narrative can reflect the intense sensory overwhelm and possible dissociation. Both trauma and the maternal transition disrupt self-narratives, requiring perinatal therapists to work with the lack of verbal coherence in a non-judgmental way. One of my clients said about her healing process: "My progress with myself in my maternal transition has been slow, hidden, internal, quiet". Her attentiveness to the particular pace and quality of her maternal transition process is reflective of a powerful assertion of her new maternal self in an embodied way. Her process of working through her trauma involved significant slowing down. The slowing down helped this client develop the sensory awareness necessary for building the somatic agency that led to her beginning assertion of her maternal embodied subjectivity. Themes related to sensations, pace, agency, and authority are important to invite exploration of, especially the sensory qualities of self-narratives.

The combination of sensory awareness and sensory vocabulary helps the therapist and client explore maternal bodyfulness themes. Identifying and exploring positive and negative embodied experiences of new maternal subjectivity are necessary for a mother's assertion of her maternal body identity. It is from this sense of maternal subjectivity that a mother can begin to resist and oppose the cultural narratives of patriarchal motherhood and intensive mothering (see Table 6.3 for an overview of maternal bodyfulness themes and related reflection questions).

TABLE 6.3 Themes and Reflection Questions for Cultivating Maternal Bodyfulness

Themes	Reflection Questions
Identifying and exploring positive and negative embodied experiences of new maternal subjectivity	How do you experience mothering in your body? What are some of the most positive experiences of mothering? How do they feel in your body? What are some of the most difficult experiences of mothering? How do they feel in your body?
Exploration and assertion of new maternal body identity through maternal body narratives	How does your way of mothering reflect who you are? What does it feel like in your body when you feel you are mothering in your own way?
Uncoupling power dynamics and oppressive narratives of patriarchal motherhood from the body	When do you feel that your way of mothering is your very own? How does it feel in your body when you mother in your own way, without anyone interfering or putting any expectations on you?

References

Baraitser, L. (2009). *Maternal encounters: The ethics of interruptions*. Routledge.

Beck C.T. (2017). The anniversary of birth trauma: A metaphor analysis. *The Journal of Perinatal Education*, 26(4), 219–228. 10.1891/1058-1243.26.4.219

Bernard, W.T., & Bernard, C. (1998). Passing the torch: A mother and daughter reflect on their experiences across generations. *Canadian Woman Studies/Les Cahiers De La Femme*, 18(2). Retrieved from https://cws.journals.yorku.ca/index.php/cws/article/view/8530

Caldwell, C.M. (2016). Body identity development: Definitions and discussions. *Body, Movement and Dance in Psychotherapy*, 11(4), 220–234. 10.1080/17432979.2016.1145141

Caldwell, C.M. (2018a). *Bodyfulness. Somatic practices for presence, empowerment, and waking up in this life*. Shambala.

Caldwell, C.M. (2018b). Body identity development: Who we are and who we become. In C.M. Caldwell, & L.B. Leighton (Eds.), *Oppression and the body. Roots, resistance, and resolutions* (pp. 31–50). North Atlantic Books.

de Marneffe, D. (2004). *Maternal desire: On children, love, and the inner life*. Time Warner Book Group.

Granner, J.R., & Seng, J.S. (2021). Using theories of posttraumatic stress to inform perinatal care clinician responses to trauma reactions. *Journal of Midwifery & Women's Health*, 66(5), 567–578. 10.1111/jmwh.13287

Harrang, C., Tillotson, D., & Winters, N.C. (2022). General introduction. In C. Harrang, D. Tillotson, & N.C. Winters (Eds.), *Body as psychoanalytic object. Clinical applications from Winnicott to Bion and beyond* (pp. 1–9). Routledge. 10.4324/9781003195559

Hill, D. (2015). *Affect regulation theory. A clinical model*. Norton.

Hoekzema, E., van Steenbergen, H., Straathof, M., Beekmans, A., Freund, I.M., Pouwels, P.J.W., & Crone, E.A. (2022). Mapping the effects of pregnancy on resting state brain activity, white matter microstructure, neural metabolite concentrations and grey matter architecture. *Nature Communications*, 13(1), 6931. 10.1038/s41467-022-33884-8

Iyengar, U., Rajhans, R., Fonagy, P., Strathearn, L., & Kim, S. (2019). Unresolved trauma and reorganization in mothers: Attachment and neuroscience perspectives. *Frontiers in Psychology, 10*, 110. 10.3389/fpsyg.2019.00110

Johnson, K.A. (2021). *Call of the wild: How we heal trauma, awaken our own power, and use it for good.* Harper Wave.

Kuhfuß, M., Maldei, T., Hetmanek, A., & Baumann, N. (2021). Somatic experiencing – effectiveness and key factors of a body-oriented trauma therapy: A scoping literature review. *European Journal of Psychotraumatology, 12*, 1929023. 10.1080/20008198.2021.1929023

LaPierre, A. (2015). Relational body psychotherapy (or relational somatic psychology). *International Body Psychotherapy Journal, 14*(2), 80–100.

Levine, P.A. (2010). *In an unspoken voice. How the body releases trauma and restores goodness.* North Atlantic Books.

Levine, P.A., Blakeslee, A., & Sylvae, J. (2018). Reintegrating fragmentation of the primitive self: Discussion of "Somatic Experiencing", *Psychoanalytic Dialogues, 28*(5), 620–628, 10.1080/10481885.2018.1506216

Orbach, S. (2006). How can we have a body?: Desires and corporeality. *Studies In Gender & Sexuality, 7*(1), 89–111.

Orbach, S. (2009). *Bodies.* Picador.

Orbach, S. (2011). Losing Bodies. *Social Research, 78*(2), 387–394.

Parker, R. (1995). *Mother love/mother hate.* BasicBooks.

Phillips, J. (2022). *The baby on the fire escape. Creativity, motherhood, and the mind-baby problem.* W.W. Norton & Company.

Piccini, O. (2021). The mother's body, the role of pleasure in the mother–infant relationship, and the traumatic risk. *International Forum of Psychoanalysis, 30*(3), 129–138. 10.1080/0803706X.2021.1946140

Porges, S.W. (2022). Polyvagal theory: A science of safety. *Frontiers in Integrative Neuroscience, 16*, 871227. 10.3389/fnint.2022.871227

Price, C.J., & Hooven, C. (2018). Interoceptive awareness skills for emotion regulation: Theory and approach of mindful awareness in body-oriented therapy (MABT). *Frontiers in Psychology, 9*, 798. 10.3389/fpsyg.2018.00798

Rutherford, H.J., Wallace, N.S., Laurent, H.K., & Mayes, L.C. (2015). Emotion regulation in parenthood. *Developmental Review: DR, 36*, 1–14. 10.1016/j.dr.2014.12.008

Schore, A.N. (2021). The interpersonal neurobiology of intersubjectivity. *Frontiers in Psychology, 12*, 648616. 10.3389/fpsyg.2021.648616

Selvam, R. (2022). *The practice of embodying emotions. A guide for improving cognitive, emotional, and behavioral outcomes.* North Atlantic Books.

Simkin, P., & Klaus, P. (2004). *When survivors give birth: Understanding and healing the effects of early sexual abuse on childbearing women.* Classic Day Publishing.

Strathearn, L., Li, J., Fonagy, P., & Montague, P.R. (2008). What's in a smile? Maternal brain responses to infant facial cues. *Pediatrics, 122*(1), 40–51. 10.1542/peds.2007-1566

7

Expansion and Integration
Trauma Release During the Perinatal Period

The Nature and Timing of Somatic Trauma Treatment

The initial and most important step of any trauma healing is to establish safety, relationally and somatically. The foundational work of building sensory awareness is a prerequisite for processing traumatic memories because it establishes the necessary amount of nervous system stability. Unfortunately, an understanding of trauma treatment has developed that separates this foundational work from "focused trauma processing". From this understanding, the slow-paced work of establishing therapeutic rapport, learning about the biopsychosocial impact of trauma through psychoeducation, and practicing tools of sensory awareness are perceived as not being the main ingredients of trauma treatment. Johnson (2021) argues that a culture of addiction to intensity has developed in society stipulating that healing requires pushing beyond and "going harder". This is an unhelpful attitude that creates a narrow understanding of trauma healing and contributes to unrealistic and incorrect expectations for clients. The perinatal woman who is overwhelmed by her trauma-related stress is understandably desperate for relief. If she is presented with an attitude of distinguishing between the initial work of stabilizing and the intense work of targeting traumatic memories, she might feel rushed to get to the latter part that promises relief. Or worse, she might feel discouraged to begin treatment at all. I have experienced many clients expressing an understandable urge to "get it over with", thinking they must get through the hard parts of talking through the details of trauma to heal from it. A common example is the mother who had a traumatic birth and expects that the main focus of her treatment should be to dissect the birth experience. For many clients, especially if they are only a few months postpartum, focusing only on the birth experience can cause overwhelm and anxiety that isn't conducive to their healing.

I believe we must challenge clinical thinking that separates trauma processing from the work of stabilizing. If we appreciate trauma beyond its symptomology as a profound destabilization of the self, it follows that trauma healing is a process of stabilizing or re-stabilizing the self. The initial focus in somatic trauma therapy on stabilizing through therapeutic safety and regulation with sensory awareness is therefore not a form of "warm up"; it lies at the heart of trauma healing. The states of fluid body-ego boundaries that characterize the perinatal period (Balsam, 2012; Furman, 1994) make mothers vulnerable to emotional distress and overwhelm. A mother's self-protective impulses for her own organism's survival are intertwined with her impulses to protect the baby. The mother's identification with the baby has a reactive somatic component where threats to the baby's body can be experienced as threats to oneself. I believe this can also happen in the other direction, where a mother might experience threats towards herself as directly impacting her baby. Our usual understanding of the survival impulses must therefore be adjusted for the perinatal woman. The somatic identification with and coregulatory connection with the baby's nervous system makes the mother vulnerable to feelings of helplessness and powerlessness. Perinatal trauma work must prioritize working with this vulnerability by both acknowledging it as a necessary part of the maternal transition and supporting the mother in orienting to her sense of agency and relative safety.

When receiving trauma treatment, clients can experience a temporary worsening of symptoms and overwhelm. This is particularly difficult for the new mother who is in a logistically challenging position for starting psychotherapy, in addition to her emotional vulnerability. The worsening of dysregulation symptoms can be mitigated and prevented with psychoeducation, emphasizing stabilization with sensory awareness, slowing down, and avoiding activating narrating traumatic events. Mothers need reassurance that treatment that initially does not focus on intense narrating or processing of traumatic events is still effective treatment that will eventually lead to healing. Trauma treatment for mothers should not follow treatment models developed for non-mothers; it must be formed around the daily reality of mothering and the psychological vicissitudes of the maternal transition. We must adapt our clinical conceptualization and treatment planning to this reality.

The Cyclical Nature of Maternal Trauma Healing

The maternal transition has an embedded element of depression broadly understood as a psychological struggle of loss, grief, and growth. The creativity of the new maternal identity carries a shadow of the loss of the pre-motherhood self that is forever lost. But the mother carries her pre-motherhood self on an emotional level, and this part is engaged in her healing process by connecting to the life-long development of her sensory awareness and regulatory capacities. Healing of trauma in the perinatal period is different; it is not a neat and linear process where symptoms are targeted and resolved, and the client then moves on. Consider that perinatal trauma reactions can be delayed (see the section on delayed onset in Introduction to Part II). The nature of perinatal trauma makes the healing process an intertwined part of the mother's adjustment to her new maternal identity and her family dynamics. The demands of mothering are unrelenting and cannot be paused. A woman's reproductive life journey continues. This can be a challenge, but it can also be clinically appreciated as part of the dynamic.

A mother will experience ebbs and flows in her growing attachment and bonding with her child as she is processing a traumatic childbirth in the months and years after giving birth. A woman who experienced a pregnancy loss will be reworking this trauma during her continued journey to conceive where opportunities for deepening her healing as well as activation and reminders of the trauma will occur. The emotional impact of fertility treatment might not be fully realized and accessible for processing until after a baby is born. For traumatic childbirth, the anniversary of the birth is a central activation point (Beck, 2017). Balsam (2012) has pointed out that women think about their births and other reproductive life events years before and after they occur. Perinatal trauma treatment should therefore adopt a slowed-down and gentle process with long-term perspectives. However, this should not be paternalistically motivated; that we must not activate a mother too much because it might influence her mothering. The gentle pace is for the mother's sake, based on an appreciation of how the trauma-healing process intertwines with the maternal journey and therefore cannot be rushed. We must work to both integrate the way mothering interacts with the trauma healing process and support women in claiming the importance of their healing process, so it doesn't "drown" in the demands of family life. Especially for developmental trauma, the healing process towards resilience is time-consuming and requires significant patience (Kain & Terrell, 2018).

In Caldwell's (2018) concept of bodyfulness, the physical realities of both past and future are acknowledged through the body "as it occupies the present moment" (p. 163). In maternal development, the narratives of past and future self are connected through the maternal embodiment of the present moment; the way one's current life stage connects to the lifelong reproductive journey through the body. The healing process in the maternal transition is inevitably intertwined with the bodily destabilization and re-stabilization of the self. Body narratives of the perinatal period are unique because the understanding of what delineates the self undergoes a reframing, a destabilization of subjectivity. Cultivating a sense of maternal bodyfulness is a way to connect to the pre-motherhood and future selves through the life-long reproductive body story. It is important to distinguish between the layers of trauma in the mother's life story, for example, new-onset trauma directly related to the birth versus chronic trauma from childhood maltreatment that was re-activated by the birth (Acton et al., 2015). Trauma treatment that goes beyond symptom reduction depends on a life-span perspective where themes of releasing traumatic overwhelm, integration of experiences, and expansion of experiential capacity and affect tolerance are bodyfully re-visited, meaning they are explored with a continued focus on sensory and experiential aspects and reflective responsiveness to these sensations.

Releasing Maternal Trauma Through Expansion of Experiential Capacity

The somatic resolution of trauma symptoms comes from changing interoceptive and proprioceptive sensations associated with the traumatic experience so that freeze responses are uncoupled from overwhelming fear and subsequently processed by completion of the nervous system activation cycle (Kuhfuß et al., 2021; Levine, 2010). The primary goal is to modify the stress response to the trauma by firstly helping the client increase tolerance for the arousal associated with the trauma with internal and external resources of sensory awareness, and secondly to guide the client carefully through a release process that facilitates the completion of the nervous system survival response (Levine, 2010).

However, the somatic approach alone does not account for the psychological conditions of motherhood. A psychoanalytic and matricentric feminist understanding of trauma healing appreciates the improvement in nervous system functioning and completion of survival responses in the context of the maternal body narrative and maternal identity formation. When survival responses are processed and completed, they contribute to a mother's experiential assertion of her embodied maternal subjectivity. The sensory overwhelm of traumatic stress instigates a feeling of fragmentation that intertwines with the inherent destabilizing of the self that motherhood entails. The reintegration of the self in the healing of perinatal trauma cannot be separated from the process of claiming maternal subjectivity. This is a process that builds from sensory awareness and is supported by coregulatory attunement. Perinatal trauma healing is therefore not only the release of trauma dysregulation patterns, but also the coregulatory integration of this release as a central part of the embodied maternal identity transformation.

Because of the intertwining of trauma healing and the maternal transition, the emergence of the embodied experience of the maternal self has a victorious or triumphant quality in the context of healing. When the mother experiences progress in her healing, she also experiences the victory of claiming her hard-earned new maternal self and her unique way of mothering. This victory reflects the empowerment that comes from claiming one's mothering as an embodied expression of self, in opposition to the pressure of motherhood as an external culturally prescribed role. When a mother experiences a release of traumatic psychic material in the context of her maternal development, this resolution becomes embedded in her bodily process of mothering, which then becomes a form of victory over the bodylessness caused by patriarchal motherhood. The empowerment of trauma healing in the perinatal context will inevitably stimulate empowered mothering. The maternal transition and the experience of trauma both involve a process of coming undone, and they also both hold the potential for the healing experience of coming back into wholeness. My assertion is that these potentials cannot be separated.

But the reintegration into wholeness necessitates a relational experience of coregulation. It is the relational aspect of trauma healing that expands the mother's experiential capacity. The coregulatory expansion of the therapeutic relationship is stimulated by the parallel development of the mother's coregulatory relationship with her baby. When we prioritize sitting with and experiencing the dysregulation of our client in the perinatal transferential field, we work to reframe the negative associations of her dysregulation as intolerable and unwanted to an understanding of her dysregulation as something that cannot be separated from her adjustments to motherhood and therefore should not be unduly pathologized. We also reframe the dysregulation as valuable nonverbal communication of relational information acknowledged through resonance and somatic transference. The somatic dysregulation and emotional states of fragmentation are reframed as components of the journey to claim the expanded sense of the maternal self. Healing perinatal trauma is thus not seen as the resolution of a negative experience, but as the development of new relational nervous system capacities in the service of assertion of maternal subjectivity.

The *Somatic Maternal Healing* approach is expansive rather than segmental (see Figure 7.1). The foundation of stabilizing and establishing safety continues throughout the treatment process. When the client's tolerance for sensations and affects is increased, internal and external regulating resources can be identified and practiced, for example, grounding through sensory awareness, orienting to the environment, and proprioceptive engagement. This foundation of stability and regulating resources are instrumental to the client's gradual integration and release of trauma memories and affects through slowly shifting between different sensations and states. The release of traumatic stress is aligned with the increase in the client's experiential capacity and her assertion of her maternal embodied subjectivity. When the client can experience the sensations and feelings related to trauma memories without being overwhelmed by dysregulation, the charge from fight, flight, and freeze responses can be discharged and nervous system activation cycles can be completed, leading to the expansion of experiential capacity.

Just as the sense of self is expanded by the maternal transition, the healing of perinatal trauma is a process of expansion. But this process must be supported by the therapist's engagement with somatic transference dynamics. The therapist must be willing to somatically receive the client's experience of destabilization (Orbach, 2006). The re-stabilization of the self is thus a coregulatory process. Levine (2010) contends that a hallmark of

Expansion and
integration

Gradual integration of
traumatic memories

Build internal and
external resources
through bodyfulness

Increase affect
tolerance with
sensory
awareness

Stabilizing &
safety

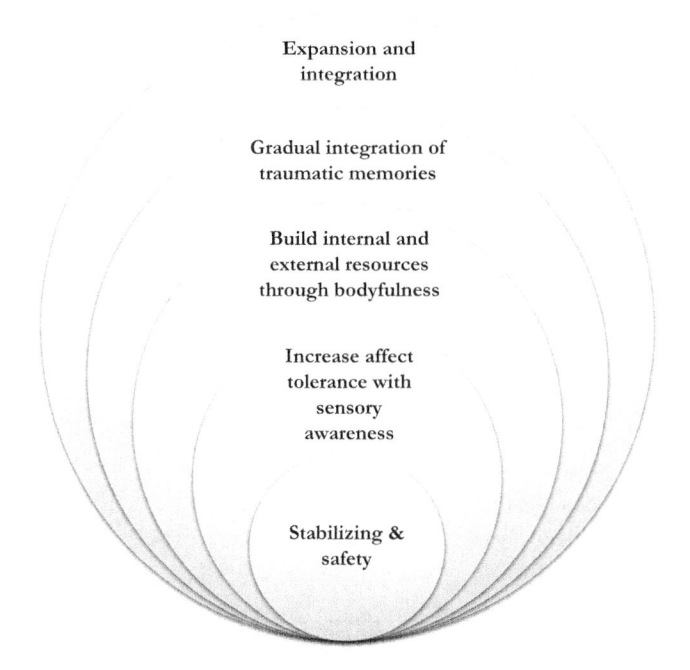

FIGURE 7.1 Expansive Model of Somatic Maternal Healing

trauma healing is to resolve the over-coupling of immobility and fear that the trauma caused so the feeling of aliveness can be restored. In the context of perinatal trauma healing, this process should not only be supported by a coregulating therapist, but a somatically *shared* experience of coming into aliveness through attunement.

Using Sensory Awareness Skills to Process Traumatic Memories

Many clients find it counterintuitive or impossible to explore their sensations related to traumatic memories. But discovering and exploring positive sensations and memories from before and after traumatic events is crucial as it helps to restore a full sensational picture (Levine, 2010). The intensity of the negative affects and sensations from a traumatic memory tends to drown out the neutral and positive experiences. The pleasant sensations contradict the traumatic overwhelm and facilitate neurological habituation regulation and completion of nervous system reactions (Levine et al., 2018). The essence of trauma healing lies in the restoration of a sense of aliveness (Levine, 2010) and a reconnection to full-body sensory awareness (Selvam, 2022). This aligns with the expansion of the embodied and sensory sense of self in the maternal transition.

Intrusive or re-experiencing memories, the cardinal symptom of PTSD, are some of the hardest trauma symptoms to work with. They indicate high levels of traumatic stress for the client and are extremely challenging for the new mother to experience while mothering. An advantage of working somatically is that the client is first guided to establish sensory awareness of positive or stabilizing sensations before exploring negative or unpleasant sensations, including those related to trauma. In this way, the client is helped in establishing sensations as crucial internal resources for affect tolerance and regulation so as to prevent overwhelm when processing traumatic memories (Brom et al. 2017; Levine, 2010). This means that sensory awareness practice initially does not focus on moments of flashbacks. When sensory awareness skills have been taught (see Chapter 5), the client can begin to practice implementing them as an immediate tool for responding to flashbacks. Working somatically with flashbacks requires practicing sensory awareness skills both in response to them and when they are not occurring. In Table 7.1, steps for applying the sensory awareness skills for flashbacks are presented with client instructions for each step. This exercise requires that the client is familiar with the foundations of sensory awareness skills reviewed in Chapter 5. The exercise can also be used for other forms of feeling states that do not present as flashbacks, but manifest as dysregulation themes.

Working with Specific Forms of Perinatal Trauma

Traumatic Childbirth

Traumatic childbirth is a highly activating topic. It is concretely different things for different clients and must therefore always

TABLE 7.1 Sensory Awareness Skills for Flashbacks

Step	Instructions
Observe the intrusive memory.	*Recognize that a flashback is happening. Say it out loud or internally or make a sound, gesture, or movement to express that you recognize what is happening.*
Orient with senses, identify things in the immediate surroundings.	*Regardless of how intense the memory is, keep noticing your immediate surroundings. Where are you, what is going on, what concrete environment are you in right now.*
Track interoception and exteroception.	*Notice what you are sensing in your body. If it feels intolerable, return to noticing your surroundings. If you can tolerate focusing on your internal sensations, bring your awareness to them and pause. If you feel the surroundings are overwhelming, bring your awareness to the most stable part of your body. Locate where you feel the least tension internally and focus on it.*
Shift attention to downregulate and connect to felt sense of agency.	*If either feels overwhelming, shift your attention back and forth between them and notice the difference. Notice if this movement changes your state.*
Proprioceptive engagement: Movement, shifting of posture, or self-touch combined with word or sound.	*Notice any impulse to move, shift your posture, place your hands anywhere on yourself, or make any sounds. Explore your impulses to move and go with them. If you have already done it without thinking about it, notice what it feels like. Notice if you feel any impulse to say a calming word or make a sound, for example humming.*
Settling: Track sensations of overwhelm subsiding.	*When the dysregulation from the intrusive memory begins to settle, track this in smallest possible increments. If you felt your anxiety was at a 10 out of 10 and is now at 9, notice this difference and how it manifests, for example lessening of muscle tension or slowing of breath and heart rate. When noticing any settling, remind yourself that flashbacks and panic attacks always settle, they are temporary.*

be clarified while the therapist is paying close attention to their own biases and countertransference reactions, without rushing the mother to provide details about the concrete events of the delivery. Some women associate traumatic childbirth with "hospital preterm emergency c-section delivery and NICU stay" while others think of "having to fight with insensitive and intrusive providers during labor". Traumatic childbirth is a form of trauma that shows the layered nature of perinatal trauma as it is hard to isolate the traumatic childbirth experience from the other aspects of the maternal transition. While the client experiences the delivery as the main traumatic event, the stress leading up to and in the immediate aftermath are crucial factors. The immediate meaning-making of the delivery experience influences how the birth is processed. Lack of attunement or defensive attitudes from providers and family can contribute to the mother's experience of trauma.

The inherent hypervigilance of the postpartum state combined with the added layers of stress from a traumatic delivery experience can make the new mother appear hypomanic, obsessive, and highly dysregulated, or numb, shut down, and dissociated. Clinicians must make a dedicated effort to prevent and internally address their judging of a mother's rumination related to her birth, especially their somatic reactions. It is impossible for a mother to refrain from making profound meanings of her birth experience whether it was traumatic or not. Birth is a transcendent and life-changing event that touches deep into a woman's sense of self, spirituality, and unconscious. While it is our job as clinicians to help our clients understand the dysregulation symptoms of trauma-related ruminations and how to change them with somatic self-regulation skills, we must never judge a mother's attachment to the meaning of her birth experience. As with all meaning-making, the meanings related to a birth experience will change and be reframed over time through healing and new life experiences. We can offer the hope that the negative meanings of a traumatic birth experience can change profoundly through healing, but this is often a long-term process that can take years. Long before a mother can reach such a goal of reframing the negative beliefs and meanings associated with a traumatic birth, she must work to lessen the activation and dysregulation related to the traumatic memory of it. The desire to reframe the negative meanings first is understandable, but the efforts are futile if the cognitive reframing is done without nervous system regulation.

From a regulation perspective of reducing overwhelm, it can be helpful to change between addressing the birth trauma itself and working on the somatic coregulation experiences of mothering. Establishing a felt experience of relative safety is crucial to help the mother reorient to the present moment when flashbacks or ruminations send her nervous system into a state of high alert. Traumatic childbirth is characterized by feeling stripped of one's dignity, feeling not cared for, that providers failed to communicate appropriately, feelings of powerlessness, exposure, and lack of control, having one's experience be dismissed or ignored, feeling abandoned, betrayed, and lonely, and feeling disconnected from the baby and partners (Beck et al., 2013). Threats to oneself and to the baby become intertwined during and immediately following delivery where the mother has not fully processed the bodily separation from the baby. She might experience somatically that any danger to her baby is a danger to herself and vice versa. The therapeutic work of reestablishing a sense of relative safety must therefore be connected to the emotional and somatic bond with the baby.

Pregnancy and Infant Loss

Giannandrea and colleagues (2013) have pointed out that pregnancy loss interacts with other trauma. Dates and temporal themes are salient for pregnancy and infant loss. The original due date of a lost pregnancy or a prematurely born infant who did not survive, reaching a gestational milestone in a new pregnancy that marked the ending of a previous one, birthdays of infants who died; these can be strong trauma reminders that the mother may or may not be prepared for. Even when a mother is rationally aware of an upcoming date that carries significance, she might not be prepared for its emotional and somatic activation. The reminders of pregnancy and infant loss can easily be overlooked by the surroundings, causing feelings of loneliness.

A lost baby, whether unborn, stillborn, or lost in infancy, is a unique grief unlike any other. The baby embodies the destabilization of the mother's subjectivity; the baby is her own emerging being, yet still intertwined with the mother, physically and psychologically. It is thus a confusing web to grieve both the parts of oneself psychologically and somatically invested in and identified with the baby, and the actual baby as a separate person and their short physical presence in the mother's life. The maternal transition entails a psychobiological process of shifting body boundaries where the mother's process of investing in her child as a bodily part of herself gradually releases as the child's development unfolds (Furman, 1994). In the case of pregnancy or infant loss, this process is short-circuited. The bereaved mother cannot go through the usual slow experience in her body of the delicate process of letting go of the part of herself that was invested in the baby. The grieving process is deeply complex in its intertwining of parts of self and parts of the baby that were not fully integrated yet. The imagined baby can continue to grow in the psyche of the mother, for example through ongoing meaning-making of the baby's role in the family story or through spiritual reflections. It is important to refrain from pathologizing such projections, especially if they help the mother grieve by pronouncing the baby's form as an independent subject that is more accessible to differentiation and mourning.

Mothers who experienced loss often present with sensations of emptiness and a sense of somatic confusion about what was lost. It can feel difficult to identify the sensations related to the loss as the body is the site of the loss. For some mothers, it can be helpful to distinguish between the feelings, sensations, and body states related to the traumatic memories (the concrete shocking events surrounding the loss) and those related to the loss of the baby's presence in their life. These themes can be worked with somatically by locating and differentiating between sensations and body states of loss and the experiences of stability, safety, and attunement. Supporting the client in identifying and tracking her shifts between these states cultivates sensory awareness and somatic agency and helps to integrate the experiences of loss. The emotions of loss are thus embodied by more parts of the body, so they become more bearable and accessible for regulation (Selvam, 2022). The goal is not to eliminate the feelings and body states related to loss, but to integrate them as tolerated components of the mother's reproductive body narrative so their somatic activation is reduced.

Childhood Maltreatment and Abuse

A starting point for developmental trauma work is to assess the degree of insight and self-observer capacity of the client and how the maternal transition has impacted this. The degree to which the birth of a baby impacts a mother's nervous system self-awareness varies greatly. A high level of cognitive insight pre-motherhood about developmental trauma and attachment-related dysregulation patterns does not always correspond with somatic self-awareness in the postpartum. It is important that the therapist verbally and nonverbally reflects back curiosity about how the mother's attachment system has been changed by the birth of the baby. In other words, we should not ask a client *if* she her attachment and regulation systems have been impacted by motherhood, but rather *how*.

Somatic receptivity and coregulation are central themes when working with developmental trauma and can be topics to explore the client's somatic self-awareness with. The client's somatic relationship with receiving support (somatic receptivity) can be simultaneously explored in explicit reflective ways and implicit through examination of the perinatal transferential field using resonance (see Chapter 5). Working with attachment trauma healing elicits deep expressions of transferential dynamics (Kain & Terell, 2018). Perinatal therapists must pay special attention to the somatic transferential dynamics and barriers to somatic receptivity for the client. Somatic transference dynamics can be elicited by sensory awareness exercises. The client can for example experience that new uncomfortable interoceptive information is caused by the therapist (Kain & Terell, 2018). The client might respond negatively towards the therapist when tracking sensations and interoceptive shifts and express a sense of a power struggle. Such an external locus of control perspective is a common somatic transference dynamic in developmental trauma (Kain & Terell, 2018).

Kain and Terrell (2018) point out that clients with developmental trauma can struggle with somatic differentiation of coregulatory experiences and might be confused about whether a certain body state is coming from themselves or the therapist. The therapist must be careful to track both the client's and their own sensations and notice both alignments and differences and how they impact the therapeutic relationship. It is namely this coregulatory experience of the therapist making use of their own somatic reactions in the resonant field to inform the therapeutic interventions that constitute the antidote to the developmental trauma. Through the coregulatory tracking of the client's states and shifts, the client is helped to distinguish between somatic trauma memories of bodylessness that mothering activates and sensations of present-moment maternal bodyfulness. The new mother's assertion of her maternal subjectivity will then complement the claiming of the childhood self that was never fully claimed. The cultivating of maternal bodyfulness becomes a new embodied expression of self that had not been possible before.

Clinical Vignette: Sarah's Integration of Deadness and Aliveness

This case illustrates my client Sarah's[1] process of healing from a traumatic childbirth and a childhood with emotional abuse from a narcissistic father. The traumatic birth experience caused a significant disconnect that left her feeling dead inside. Sarah's healing process was focused on both integrating her feelings of deadness on a somatic level and discovering her new sensations of aliveness through her embodied maternal subjectivity.

Sarah was a 25-year-old married woman who gave birth to her first child, a healthy baby boy, at a planned home birth with the attendance of a midwife, a doula, an assistant, and her husband. Sarah came to therapy about 4 months after the birth and presented with symptoms of PTSD and severe depression.

She reported feeling highly anxious and shifting between states of rage, frustration, hypomania, and overwhelm, and states of despair, apathy, fatigue, numbness, and a feeling of "being dead" in her chest. She also reported having random flashbacks about the birth, and that she cut all contact with her midwife after the delivery, refusing to attend the 6-weeks follow-up. Any conversations about birth, especially in the context of the homebirth community she had been a part of during prenatal care, were very upsetting to Sarah and triggered anger and despair. At the same time, Sarah would find herself ruminating and obsessively researching medical information online about details related to birth and her experiences during delivery. This obsessive research would often happen at night on her phone, at times when she should have been sleeping.

Sarah described the birth experience as "awful" and traumatic although she stated that she and her baby were medically "fine" and that she her physical recovery had been good. Although she was happy that she was physically okay, she experienced her husband's focus on her physical health as a dismissal of her emotional struggles. Sarah described her husband as emotionally stable and generally supportive, but that she felt he did not understand her emotionally: "He means well, but he has zero idea of what it's like to give birth and all that, he just doesn't get it". Sarah described feeling deeply depressed, but it took several months of sessions before she was able to articulate the underlying shame and self-loathing that caused her low mood. Sarah had felt a contradictory mix of anger towards the midwife and towards herself, sometimes switching between the two. "Sometimes I feel like it was all her fault and I hate her, and sometimes I feel like it was all my own fault, I caused it all by myself," she said. The self-blame was a pervasive theme that seemed to be an internal tormentor for her. Sarah was in labor for about 48 hours and spend almost 4 hours in the pushing stage. He baby's heart rate was indicating increasing stress during the pushing. Sarah said she had felt lonely and abandoned during the entire birth. She described having had several moments of feeling like "they were talking behind my back" and that she did not feel communicated with.

After hours of pushing, the midwife introduced the idea of doing an episiotomy, that Sarah said she felt she did not truly consent to. She described feeling violated and betrayed, but that she did not recognize this until much later. Sarah described having been overly nice towards the birth attendants when they visited the day after the birth, but that she soon felt incapable of having any contact with them. After some months, she realized the most painful part had been the feeling of being dismissed by the midwife. Sarah described her as defensive and unwilling to acknowledge any of Sarah's feelings and "clearly in over her head with that homebirth".

Sarah was the youngest child, with 2 brothers 5 and 7 years older than her. She grew up in a suburban lower middle-class family. Her mother was a stay-at-home mother who occasionally worked part-time as a cleaning lady. Her father worked in appliance sales and would often travel. Sarah described him as a narcissist who rarely showed emotion: "He was mostly in his own world, except for when he was excited about sports or something, or if he got upset with us. Then he would explode." She described her mother as somewhat downtrodden, but with a certain amount of stoicism and resiliency that kept her rather unfazed by the father's outbursts. Sarah described that she could see her mother's strengths but that she also felt disappointed and at times enraged by her mother's lack of courage to stand up for herself. "My mom would just be quiet and go about her stuff, she never engaged when my dad was upset," Sarah stated. I was curious about Sarah's nervous system experiences in her family growing up, but she struggled to verbalize or experientially explore any memories. Sarah had felt "bored and frustrated" at home. She had never felt close to her father but learned early on to avoid him. She described feeling somewhat close to her mother and her brothers in her early childhood, but that she started feeling repulsed by her mother when she started puberty. She described her brothers as aloof and impatient with her, although at times they bonded when something exciting happened, like a birthday party or Holidays. Overall, she described her family of origin as "not very warm". Sarah had suffered from periods of depression and anxiety since her teenage years.

One of the main somatic symptoms Sarah experienced was feeling a sense of deadness in her chest; a fantasy that the flesh of her chest was dead. "It is as if that part of me is corpse," she stated. Sarah stated that she had never had this experience before the birth of her baby. We explored it in depth, and I was puzzled by the fact that she had described her breastfeeding experience as very positive with relatively few challenges that occurred mostly in the first month postpartum. She had felt pride in her good milk supply, she had enjoyed her husband's marveling at her breasts, and it had made her feel sexually attractive. She would switch between feeling positive or neutral about breastfeeding and then suddenly feeling a sense of deadness. Interestingly, she did not feel the deadness while nursing, but at other times during the day. Sarah expressed feeling bonded with her baby but described feeling that even the positive interactions with him felt "too intense". With a thorough exploration of her daily life, Sarah developed awareness of her patterns of rushing everything, including positive interactions: "I just have to keep moving, it's so hard for me to stand still". At the time, Sarah did not show any signs of health issues and was in good physical health, but several months later she developed thyroid issues. While it was not confirmed at the time, in hindsight I wonder if Sarah was experiencing subclinical thyroid issues that contributed to her dysregulation.

We spent a lot of time sitting with her somatic feelings of deadness and the sense of deep despair that came with it and exploring her sensory and affective shifts. Sarah expressed feeling a Catch-22 related to whether she should verbalize her feelings of shame or not. "The shame is too intense," she would say, "I can't stand talking about it, but if I don't talk about it, I will be swallowed by depression. But if I talk about it with anyone, they will not be able to understand and that will hurt. I am completely alone". I struggled to make sense of her contradictory states and experienced confusion in my thoughts and body. It was as if Sarah's states of depression and shame would reach a point where it became too intense for her to sense herself, causing her to shut down any sensory awareness. However, the intensity of her feelings and sensations seemed to re-appear through her anger outbursts, as forms of displacements.

During the first months of treatment, Sarah was highly sensitive to any misattunement on my part. She would express anger and frustration if I misunderstood anything or made suggestions that did not work for her. Although she did not verbalize anger towards me or confronted me directly, I had a strong feeling of her being furious with me. I noticed that my countertransference responses were most often a form of shutting down rather than feeling activated or defensive. I felt a sense of disconnect from emotions and sensations when she was angry. This was not only when she was frustrated with me, but also when she expressed anger towards others. I felt touched by her states of despair and would feel my eyes well up and my heart sink, but I felt oddly numb to her anger. She described having seen a therapist before me who had been eager to support her, but, as Sarah put it, "she was unable to deal with what I was feeling. I could just sense how uncomfortable I made her". I understood the message to me in this; that I had to prove that I was not like the previous therapist who couldn't handle her overwhelm. During many sessions, I found myself observing my own numbness as a reaction to her anger and working hard to stay connected to this observation and to track the shifts from numbness to the felt sense of resonance with Sarah's other states. I wondered about the numbness in light of Sarah's developmental history. She described feeling numb about her father's anger outbursts when we explored her childhood. At one point Sarah mentioned that although she could get very frustrated with her husband, she did like that he would try to appease her anger. "He wants to help, but he has no clue how to. But at least he doesn't shut me out like my mother did," she said. Sarah's mother had always responded with stoic indifference to any anger from Sarah or her brothers. It became clear to me that my somatic countertransference of numbness in reaction to her anger was a barrier to our work and something I had to work on. I practiced tracking any sensations thoroughly when I noticed the feeling of numbness arise to differentiate the levels of numbness and integrate more sensory awareness into the transferential field.

We continued to explore Sarah's shifting states and worked on supporting her relationship with sensations. We discovered through collaboration that she was experiencing a deep split between feelings of aliveness and deadness. Around 9 months postpartum, Sarah felt resourced and stable enough to process the birth experience. She identified sensations of connection and warmth in her arms related to the memory of holding her baby for the first time, and in contrast a complete lack of sensations in her legs. Sarah came to the realization that she had felt completely shut off from the waist and down during the delivery and that she felt fragmented by this experience of being split in half. We explored her sensory awareness of her feet and worked to re-establish a sense of connection down through her legs. She reported that pushing her feet and carefully sensing the impulse to kick seemed to help he feel more integrated. In a later session, Sarah reported feeling an impulse to kick that felt deeply satisfying. This could have been an impulse for a survival response movement that was not completed during the traumatic birth. We explored how it was understandable and necessary for Sarah to have split off her sensations in her lower body during and after the delivery and it seemed like that verbalization helped Sarah allow herself to focus on the parts that were not split off, namely her upper body and her arms where she felt strong somatic memories of the first moments of bonding with her baby. She realized the sense of stability and grounding that those sensations and images held and was able to connect them to her current bonding with her baby. While I felt an increase in our shared experience of her integration of the positive somatic memories of holding her baby, I felt an even stronger sense of resonance and invigoration from her impulses to kick. The impulse had not felt like her usual anger or rage, but a different feeling of aliveness. It seemed like we were only able to experience a new shared state of aliveness after I had shared Sarah's state of frustration and disconnect.

The shifting between the state of feeling split off, dissociated, and numb, and the state of integration and aliveness was at first experienced as very intense. Sarah would say she felt it was like two ways of functioning that were hard to reconcile.

"I had to protect my baby from all the dark feelings. He was this new life and what happened during the birth felt like a death. It felt like part of me died. I had to set up a wall between my baby and the feelings of love for him and the darkness of what happened, the death parts. I was so scared that he would feel that darkness," she said. I invited Sarah to practice tracking both the sensations related to the fear and sensations related to experiencing her bonding with her baby in the here-and-now. While I acknowledged her concern about her trauma impacting her baby, I encouraged her to focus on how she was also connecting with her baby through her aliveness. Sarah practiced this shifting when she felt overwhelmed by shame and fear of harming her baby. She discovered that getting breaks from her baby helped her deepen her sensory awareness of the positive interactions of aliveness with her baby when she was reunited with him. Sarah also wrote poems as part of her healing process, but she was unable to bring them to session or to talk about them. "It's too painful to read them. They are all about the deadness I felt, my body feeling like a corpse, it's disgusting. But it was good to get them out", she said.

By the end of her treatment, after 18 months, Sarah would talk about feeling a sense of triumph. After months of feeling angry about the thought of having sex, Sarah felt a new desire to be intimate with her husband and described it as healing. She had started exercising more and felt a tremendous sense of victory from it. It was clear that her exercise at times was done with hypomanic energy and reflected dysregulation patterns, but Sarah continued to develop insight about this. She expressed feeling aware of her life-long tendency to push herself hard and get "over-active" as a way of coping with anxiety and forcefully pushing away feelings of lethargy. She also realized that the more she felt a sense of triumph, the less activated she felt by traumatic memories. As she built a sense of confidence in her maternal body – "a body that had survived," as she said – she experienced a lessening of trauma symptoms and sympathetic arousal. She described that although she still felt wounded and sad for how her body had been violated, she also felt a sense of triumph through the aliveness she was able to connect to: "I guess feeling my body did heal after all and that I am alive despite feeling dead is a way I can have myself."

Sarah's healing process was one of high intensity emotionally and somatically. She struggled with slowing down because it was deeply painful for her: Slowing down made her feel the sense of deadness that the traumatic birth had caused, echoing body states from her developmental history with a narcissistic father whom she felt was unable to provide her a sense of coregulatory reciprocity. It was crucial for Sarah that her process of discovering her bodily sense of being split in half wasn't rushed. The invasiveness of the delivery and the relational betrayal she experienced from the midwife sent her into a state of harsh splitting off feelings of deadness from aliveness that echoed her emotional survival strategy and regulation patterns of her developmental history. Sarah's coregulation experience with her baby was challenged by this, but the compartmentalization of her feelings served her to stay partly connected to the sensory aspects of mothering. Her splitting was a powerful survival strategy that I believe helped her connect with her baby in a bodily way, even if her interactions with him were characterized by hypervigilance and at times hypomanic energy. However, the spitting could not maintain her, and the sense of deadness was pulling at her like a dark night. It felt like Sarah spent a lot of her energy staving off the deadness with her hypomanic energy, until she succumbed to it. Her shifting between these states was rigid and painful. It took a considerable amount of time for us to find a shared rhythm of moving between these states. I had to maintain faith in Sarah's capacity for shifting between states and refrain from trying to save her from her discomfort, as she also refused this with her anger towards me. I believed this anger was a significant barrier to her somatic receptivity that had to be worked through on a bodily level between us: I had to tolerate my own numbness on a self-regulatory level before I could expect Sarah to engage in the somatic transferential field. It was through this relational support that Sarah eventually learned to tolerate the discomfort of these shifts, which enabled her to develop the flexibility to move between them and have more agency in modifying them.

Working with Sarah was a collaborative work of expansion of experiential capacity by relational integration of dissociated parts. Highly intense states of aliveness had to be reconciled with a body state as ponderous as "deadness". Sarah's initiation into motherhood thrust her into the darkness of split-off body states of shut-down. I came to see her hyperarousal as much more than merely "dysregulation", but as her survival energy forcefully trying to keep the feeling of deadness at bay lest she be swallowed by it. Unconscious material surfaced through bodily sensations and states and the dynamic between them. It was through the reworking of these dynamics of bodily states that Sarah claimed her new maternal self.

Note

1 Sarah's case is de-identified and details have been changed to protect confidentiality.

References

Acton, C., Fisher, J., Rowe, H., & Taylor, J. (2015). The postnatal period – opportunities for creating change. In J. Seng, & J. Taylor (Eds.), *Trauma informed care and the perinatal period* (pp. 74–92). Dunedin Academic Press Limited.

Balsam, R.H. (2012). *Women's bodies in psychoanalysis*. Routledge. 10.4324/9780203078327

Beck, C.T. (2017). The anniversary of birth trauma: A metaphor analysis. *The Journal of Perinatal Education, 26*(4), 219–228. 10.1891/1058-1243.26.4.219

Beck, C. T., Driscoll, J. W., & Watson, S. (2013). *Traumatic childbirth* (1st ed.). Routledge. 10.4324/9780203766699.

Brom, D., Stokar, Y., Lawi, C., Nuriel-Porat, V., Ziv, Y., Lerner, K., & Ross, G. (2017). Somatic experiencing for posttraumatic stress disorder: A randomized controlled outcome study. *Journal of Traumatic Stress, 0*, 1–9. 10.1002/jts.22189

Caldwell, C.M. (2018). *Bodyfulness. Somatic practices for presence, empowerment, and waking up in this life*. Shambala.

Furman, E. (1994). Early aspects of mothering: What makes it so hard to be there to be left. *Journal of Child Psychotherapy, 20*(2), 149–164. 10.1080/00754179408256746

Giannandrea, A.M., Cerulli, C., Anson, E., & Chaudron, L.H. (2013). Increased risk for postpartum psychiatric disorders among women with past pregnancy loss. *Journal of Women's Health, 22*(9), 760–768. 10.1089/jwh.2012.4011

Johnson, K.A. (2021). *Call of the wild: How we heal trauma, awaken our own power, and use it for good.* Harper Wave.

Kain, K.L., & Terrell, S.J. (2018). *Nurturing resilience. Helping clients move forward from developmental trauma.* North Atlantic Books.

Kuhfuß, M., Maldei, T., Hetmanek, A., & Baumann, N. (2021). Somatic experiencing – effectiveness and key factors of a body-oriented trauma therapy: A scoping literature review. *European Journal of Psychotraumatology, 12,* 1929023. 10.1080/20008198.2021.1929023

Levine, P.A. (2010). *In an unspoken voice. How the body releases trauma and restores goodness.* North Atlantic Books.

Levine, P.A., Blakeslee, A., & Sylvae, J. (2018). Reintegrating fragmentation of the primitive self: Discussion of "Somatic Experiencing", *Psychoanalytic Dialogues, 28*(5), 620–628. 10.1080/10481885.2018.1506216

Orbach, S. (2006). How can we have a body?: Desires and corporeality. *Studies In Gender & Sexuality, 7*(1), 89–111.

Selvam, R. (2022). *The practice of embodying emotions. A guide for improving cognitive, emotional, and behavioral outcomes.* North Atlantic Books.

8

Making Maternal Healing Whole with Clinical Creativity and Biopsychosocial Somatic Treatment Planning

Trauma-Responsive Treatment Planning and Biopsychosocial Clinical Creativity

Perinatal treatment planning becomes trauma-responsive when it is built on the principles of trauma-informed care: Awareness of how past trauma can impact a woman's maternal transition, sensitivity to the risks of traumatization during the perinatal period, and active measures to prevent and mitigate traumatic stress reactions related to all aspects of the perinatal transition (Polmanteer et al., 2019; Seng & Taylor, 2015). A treatment model that aims to effectively treat trauma must apply a biopsychosocial approach, as trauma impacts people on biological, psychological, and social levels. Biopsychosocial clinical thinking is not so much a protocol or template as it is a reflective process. It is a philosophy of care that appreciates the client's subjective experience as an essential contributor to treatment and positions the relationship between client and provider as the starting point (Borrell-Carrió, 2004). Trauma impacts us on all levels of functioning, in intricate ways, but it is primarily a subjective experience, making it necessary to center the client's experience when conceptualizing the suffering and strategizing the treatment of it. A mother's subjective experience is central to the struggles of her maternal transition of resisting the pressures of culturally prescribed expectations for motherhood and asserting her subjectivity through her individual mothering practice.

Biopsychosocial clinical thinking about the perinatal period promotes a shift away from a pathology framework towards an appreciation of the unique potential for healing that the maternal transition brings. Identifying the correct diagnosis is only one initial step of the treatment that is processed further by the collaboration between the client and provider (Borell-Carrió, 2004). Since the relational turn of modern psychotherapy, we have come to acknowledge the uniqueness of every therapist-client dyad. In relation-focused biopsychosocial thinking, the client's role is shifted from a passive informant towards a protagonist role (Borrell-Carrió et al., 2004). In the same way, matricentric feminist philosophy acknowledges that every woman's journey of becoming a mother is a unique "reinvention" of motherhood for herself. This process of asserting a new embodied subjectivity as the place from where one mothers is a process of creativity that our clinical attitude should match. The creativity of empowered motherhood must be matched by a creative approach to treatment.

I understand clinical creativity as the experience of clinical work being a creative process between therapist and client, not only in terms of the therapeutic relationship being a unique and co-created intersubjective bond, but also in the sense of the therapeutic techniques and interventions being applied with an attitude of creativity, expansion, and flexibility. Being clinically creative is to think – and feel – in terms of theoretical flexibility, integration, connection, joyfulness, and playfulness. The clinical work becomes a creative process when theory, concepts, and clinical techniques are developed and applied beyond any protocol into something new for the unique therapeutic couple. Seemingly simple elements like referrals and practical adjustments of the therapeutic frame can be approached as ingredients of creativity. I believe therapists need to regard and engage in clinical work as something potentially creative if we are to convey an attitude of hope for healing. Clinical creativity serves many therapeutic functions, especially for cultivating intersubjective capacity, but it also offers the advantage of preventing therapist burnout. Clinical creativity is a way of cultivating the mutual pleasure of therapeutic care work that can model for a mother the importance of the bodily reward in her caretaking of her baby. When we regard the clinical process as a source of creativity, we can appreciate the joys of creativity as a form of relational reward, while attuning to the client. Even the most difficult aspects of trauma work like crisis handling, high levels of emotional pain, grief, traumatic stress, and dysregulation, can be appreciated as parts of the creative process of discovering the client's unique needs and characteristics and how they can best be met. We can take joy in witnessing and supporting a mother's discovery of her new embodied identity as a creative process.

Somatic, experiential, and expressive arts modalities are inherently creative, but clinical creativity is not only about the medium of therapy. It is just as much about the perspective and embodied mindset of the therapist. Biopsychosocial relation-focused thinking that sees the clinical process as a collaborative exploration is inherently creative. The complexity of the links between biology, psychology, and the social realm in the perinatal period poses a challenge for the mother to make sense of her maternal transition and healing process. Her discovery and claim of her new maternal embodied self is a process of struggling. The healing of working towards maternal bodyfulness can be understood as a creative struggle. In Green's (2019) research on feminist mothering, she contends that the feminist mother's assertion of her own perspective as her starting point, as opposed to defining her life from her child, makes her mothering "a dynamic place for creativity" (p. 95).

Treatment Strategy: The Maternal Bodyfulness Cycle of Empowerment

For an exploration of the treatment strategy, we must reiterate the overarching goal in *Somatic Maternal Healing:*

> To help the mother get into a mode of coregulation-supported somatically anchored reflections where she can mourn and play, process, release, and heal trauma, and eventually explore and synthesize the verbal/conscious and nonverbal/unconscious expressions of her maternal embodied and relational subjectivity. To balance the inherent vulnerability of the maternal transition with its potential for deeper healing of trauma on psychological, biological, and sociological levels, the treatment aims to support the mother in asserting her embodied subjectivity through maternal bodyfulness with:
>
> 1. Focus on supporting assertion of maternal embodied subjectivity through the perinatal-specific coregulation mode of the therapeutic relationship, sensory awareness and vocabulary, and maternal body narrative and body identity.
> 2. Anti-inflammatory measures: Psychoeducation, stress-reduction, referrals to health care providers to address inflammation-related issues like pain and auto-immune conditions, nervous system somatic work for regulation and trauma resolution.
> 3. Assertion of feminist/empowered mothering and resistance against the oppression of institutionalized patriarchal motherhood.

The biopsychosocial understanding of trauma in the perinatal context informs our treatment approach towards an increased focus on the stages of stabilization, psychoeducation, and resourcing, contributing to a strength-based attitude. We must challenge the notion from the diagnosis-focused approach that "true" trauma treatment should only consist of confrontation and intense processing of trauma memories and that the sole goal of treatment is the reduction or elimination of symptoms. Such a treatment approach is often not feasible with expecting or new mothers who are naturally emotionally, physically, and logistically limited in their treatment participation and have acute needs for reassurance and support. Their trauma symptoms might also intertwine with normal adaptations and stress reactions of the perinatal period (see Introduction to Part I for a review of trauma symptoms in the perinatal context). Because of the vulnerability of the perinatal period, the initial treatment stage of assessment and establishing rapport should be geared towards stabilization and lessening of stressors until the full clinical picture is clear. This means that intense trauma processing will rarely be advisable in the first weeks or months after birth or in the beginning stages of treatment, and for some clients, it might take even longer. From a biopsychosocial clinical approach that acknowledges the wider developmental context of trauma and the trauma healing process, these initial steps of stabilizing are still effective in the treatment of trauma. They are, in fact, necessities for subsequent deeper processing of traumatic memories. Clinical creativity that cultivates flexibility and does not rush treatment is not in opposition to treatment planning that adheres to trauma-informed care principles or medical necessity criteria but on the contrary conducive to it.

As discussed in Chapter 7, the process of trauma healing in the context of female and maternal psychological development is not linear, but involves cyclical dynamics of revisiting life stages, roles, and developmental struggles. The cycle of maternal bodyfulness mirrors the process of female adolescence where sensory awareness and body narratives lay the foundation for the assertion of the new embodied subjectivity of womanhood. The difference between experiencing empowerment and overwhelm in the maternal transition lies in an expansion of one's experiential capacity for sensory awareness and sensory vocabulary so that body narrative and body identity can be claimed and asserted in the new reality of being a mother. For mothering to be an empowered and empowering practice, it must be a bodily founded integration of the physical reality of mothering and one's adjustment to it. When mothering is experienced as empowering, the sensory aspects of it are further integrated into its personal meanings, even when it is physically intense and at times involves dysregulation. When a mother experiences chronic bodylessness, her ongoing adjustments to her maternal transition are not founded in her sensory awareness. When there is a preponderance of maternal bodyfulness, mothering becomes a reinforcing cycle of empowerment (see Figure 8.1). The treatment strategy of *Somatic Maternal Healing* is to support and reinforce the empowering cycles of maternal bodyfulness and empowered mothering through coregulatory support of sensory awareness and verbalization of maternal body narrative and identity.

Perinatal Trauma Psychoeducation

Psychoeducation is a central part of trauma treatment and reflects the trauma-informed principles of transparency,

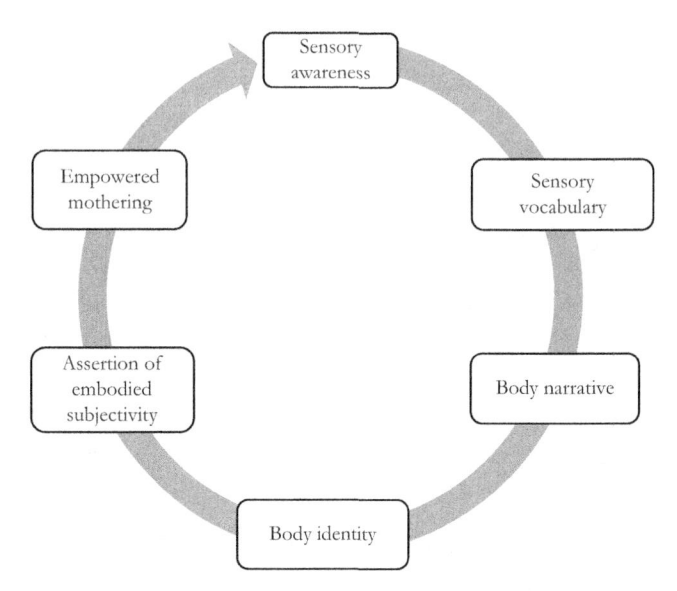

FIGURE 8.1 The Maternal Bodyfulness Cycle of Empowerment

empowerment, collaboration, and mutuality. However, learning about trauma is a nonlinear process (Johnson, 2021). Cognitive learning interacts with experiential and relational learning. For psychoeducation to be effective, it must be applied in the context of attunement and resonance and with a strong emphasis on hope. Psychoeducational content that causes overwhelm or contributes to self-blame is harmful and not therapeutic. When done right, psychoeducation may be associated with improved perinatal outcomes (Stevens et al., 2021). While our knowledge about the connections between trauma and mental health in the perinatal period is daunting, psychoeducation is founded on the premise that knowledge about the biopsychosocial dynamics of the maternal transition ultimately empowers mothers. From the affect regulation understanding of therapy as primary coregulation, psychoeducation must also be interactive. This can be done by slowing down the pace of psychoeducation and pausing to help clients connect the topic in question with relevant examples from their daily life.

The biopsychosocial widened understanding of trauma has implications for clinical language and treatment strategies. The term "trauma" is not always adequate or appropriate when working with the many layers of perinatal trauma. Too much focus on defining trauma and diagnosis can take away focus from learning about the biopsychosocial interactions and long-term effects of toxic stress and allostatic load. Effective psychoeducation maintains a continued focus on removing blame and instilling hope for healing. Furthermore, responsible trauma psychoeducation prevents and addresses overwhelm from discussing activating topics. This includes intake and assessment paperwork (see Appendix A for the perinatal intake questionnaire). The principles of attunement and resonance apply when doing psychoeducation and should be enhanced. Table 8.1. presents an overview of psychoeducation topics and their main messages.

TABLE 8.1 Topics for Psychoeducation

Psychoeducation Topics	Messages
Instilling hope and realistic expectations for healing from perinatal trauma	*Healing from postpartum depression and perinatal trauma is possible. It does require a holistic approach that addresses biological, psychological, and social aspects. Trauma treatment can be challenging in the postpartum period, but alleviation of symptoms can be achieved on a short-term basis and long-term healing continues for the rest of a person's life. Holistic treatment that focuses on self-regulation can not only reduce symptoms but also improve overall well-being.*
Widening the term "trauma" and connecting stabilizing work with trauma treatment	*Trauma can mean a lot of things to different people. We are beginning to think more broadly about trauma as we are understanding more about how it impacts our bodies and minds. Trauma can be specific events or the stress from having had a difficult childhood. Both of these impact your emotional and physical health. You don't need to have a specific trauma condition like PTSD or meet criteria for a trauma diagnosis to need and benefit from trauma-focused treatment. Trauma treatment is not only about talking through specific events or experiences. Building a safe relationship with your therapist, learning about the impact of trauma on body and mind, and learning skills of self-regulation are the foundation of trauma healing. You don't have to talk through traumatic events to be doing trauma treatment. Sometimes it can be important to not go into details about traumatic events before you are ready.*
Acknowledge the overwhelming amount of information and misinformation about PMADs and parenting	*Mothers are exposed to an abundance of information – and misinformation – about postpartum mental health and parenting. This can contribute to stress and is often unhelpful because it is generalized. For information to be helpful, it must be adjusted to the situation of the individual. A trained perinatal therapist can help you make sense of relevant information in light of your unique situation.*
Emphasize mother as authority and mothering as an individual practice	*Mothers are bombarded with parenting philosophies and ideas about the "correct" way to parent. There is no one right way of mothering. Mothering is not a performance of an objectively defined skill, but an expression of who you are, through the unique relationship between you and your child. Only you can know and decide what is the right way to mother for you. Many mothers struggle with feeling inadequate when they are exposed to social media content about parenting.*

(Cont.)

Making Maternal Healing Whole ♦ 231

TABLE 8.1 (Cont.)

Psychoeducation Topics	Messages
Shift from blame and guilt	Postpartum depression and trauma reactions involve many complex factors that are outside the control of the individual. It is not your fault. Self-blame and guilt are very common among mothers, not only those who struggle with postpartum depression or anxiety, due to unrealistic cultural expectations for mothering. Postpartum depression can be a result of underlying trauma or stress from previous life periods. Mothers and their providers are not always aware of this. Many mothers come to understand their life experiences in a new way after they become mothers.
Linking reproductive biology, Maternal Mental Health, and the vulnerability of the perinatal period	The biological changes of motherhood make us vulnerable to stress, overwhelm, and trauma. These biological factors influence our emotional and mental health. The combination of the transition to motherhood and trauma strains the nervous system. It is not a mother's fault if she experiences trauma- and stress-reactions in relation to pregnancy, delivery, and postpartum.
Anti-inflammatory measures like pain management and sleep protection	Inflammation is the body's response to stress. Because of the complex links between the biology of motherhood and stress and trauma, it is important to target all forms of inflammation, including medical issues and stress patterns. We do this by addressing any pain issues, working to protect sleep and reduce stress, and referring to relevant health care providers. Stress-reduction from psychotherapy and other forms of social support also help target inflammation.
Reframing of negative associations with sensations	It is understandable to have developed a negative relationship with sensations if you have experienced trauma or stress in your life. It is also common for new mothers to struggle with all the new sensations of mothering. But this can be changed with treatment that focuses on practicing sensory awareness. This is especially important in the transition to motherhood where one's relationship with sensations and the body undergoes big changes. If you struggle with feeling overwhelmed by the sensations of motherhood, you can learn to regulate yourself to feel better. With good support, everyone has the capacities for improving their self-regulation skills. When you develop awareness of your sensations and find new ways of coping with them, you can build your confidence and sense of self in your new identity as a mother.

Referral Considerations for Anti-Inflammatory Care

As reviewed in Chapter 2, the dynamics of trauma, toxic stress, allostatic load, inflammation, reproductive biology, and PMADs call for anti-inflammatory interventions. Research indicates that trauma-informed treatment must include an element of anti-inflammatory intervention, especially stress reduction (Gill et al., 2020; Kendall-Tackett, 2010). Referrals based on a holistic understanding of trauma and the role of inflammation must be made in the context of psychoeducation and collaboration. See Figure 8.2 for areas of anti-inflammatory interventions to consider for referrals. For the role of diet and nutritional deficiencies, standard primary care and obstetric guidelines might not be sufficient for complicated conditions related to trauma-induced stress and allostatic load. Further assessment for example with functional medicine could reveal important information related to inflammatory complications but is not accessible to all clients. It is also important to consider co-morbid eating disorders or disordered eating as possible interacting factor. Chronic or acute pain should be immediately targeted with perinatal physical therapy or lactation support to address the root cause, combined with psychoeducation on the interactions between pain, trauma, and mood (see Introduction to Part I, the section on negative mood and cognitions). When exploring resources for lifestyle changes for stress reduction, it is crucial to conceptualize it beyond individual therapy. Stress reduction for the new mother must be framed as a family and community task. The initial therapeutic conversation around stress reduction should focus on identifying individuals and community resources around the mother who can be engaged, including family involvement, community organizations, social worker support, activism and advocacy groups, peer support groups, volunteer support, and relevant faith community support. This process of compiling resources and referring to anti-inflammatory interventions can be undertaken with a creative mindset.

Figure 8.2 diagram

Center: **Anti-Inflammatory Interventions**

Surrounding nodes:
- Diet and nutritional deficiencies
- Exercise, sleep, lifestyle, stress reduction
- Pain management and physical recovery
- Treatment of PMADs and trauma causing dysregulation
- Assessing and treating medical conditions
- Social relational support

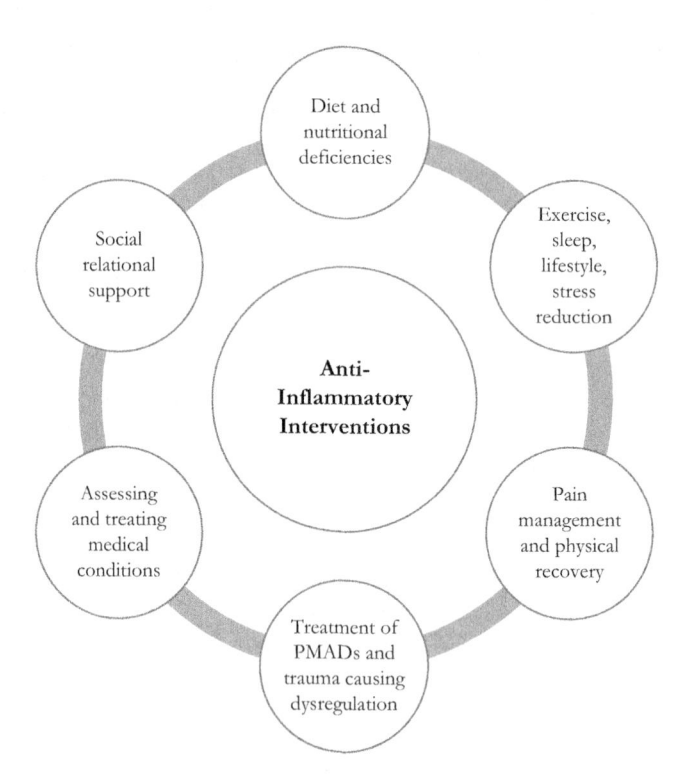

FIGURE 8.2 Referral Considerations for Anti-Inflammatory Care

Treatment Goals and Objectives

Given the importance of establishing therapeutic safety and stability in the initial stage of treatment, it is central to distinguish between and work with short-term and long-term treatment goals. As discussed, the short-term focus on stabilizing should not be minimized. The stabilization focus on the short-term goals continues throughout the course of treatment and can be revisited as needed when new life stressors emerge. In Table 8.2, short-term and long-term goals are presented, listed in the areas of biological, psychological, social, and trauma-specific. Because they are general guidelines, they should be adjusted for the individual's particular needs.

TABLE 8.2 Short-Term and Long-Term Treatment Goals

Areas	Short-Term Goals	Long-Term Goals
Biological/ somatic	♦ Identify and address issues of inflammation and acute stress with referrals for anti-inflammatory care. ♦ Identify and increase activities that promote stabilizing, relaxation, rewarding aspects of mothering. ♦ Learn and practice foundations of sensory awareness skills.	♦ Replace inflammation-inducing patterns related to health behavior and lifestyle with anti-inflammatory habits. ♦ Develop consistent habits of self-regulation with somatic regulation skills. ♦ Improve coregulatory functioning; ability to regulate from social support.
Psychological	♦ Identify and clarify main stress triggers related to subjective experience of maternal transition. ♦ Understand how personal history is interacting with maternal transition through trauma psychoeducation and exploration of developmental history. ♦ Identify positive experiences of bonding with baby and others, at any level/frequency/ capacity.	♦ Connect and integrate new maternal identity and sensory awareness. ♦ Identify and cultivate empowering practices of mothering. ♦ Cultivate rewarding experiences of mothering.
Social	♦ Identify values and priorities for new maternal identity distinguished from expectations from others. ♦ Distinguish between values/priorities from self and from others and society. ♦ Identify and engage with individuals and groups that can provide social support.	♦ Identify and assert individual style of mothering outside of cultural expectations. ♦ Develop awareness of strengths for addressing and challenging cultural expectations for mothering. ♦ Develop habits of balanced support-seeking from relevant others.

(Cont.)

TABLE 8.2 (Cont.)

Areas	Short-Term Goals	Long-Term Goals
Trauma-specific	♦ Understand the type of perinatal trauma through psychoeducation and collaboratory review of developmental and reproductive history. ♦ Identify and reduce main triggers/reminders of traumatic stress. ♦ Learn and practice somatic self-regulation skills in response to traumatic memories and dysregulation.	♦ Change dysregulation patterns related to traumatic memories with somatic self-regulation skills. ♦ Replace issues of bodily disconnect (numbing, dissociation, negativity towards body) with continued practicing of connecting sensory awareness with sense of self. ♦ Connect empowering aspects of mothering with ongoing trauma-healing.

References

Borrell-Carrió, F., Suchman, A.L., & Epstein, R.M. (2004). The biopsychosocial model 25 years later: Principles, practice, and scientific inquiry. *Annals of Family Medicine, 2*(6), 576–582. 10.1370/afm.245

Gill, H., El-Halabi, S., Majeed, A., Gill, B., Lui, L.M.W., Mansur, R.B., ... Rosenblat, J.D. (2020). The association between adverse childhood experiences and inflammation in patients with major depressive disorder: A systematic review. *Journal of Affective Disorders, 272*, 1–7. 0.1016/j.jad.2020.03.145

Green, F.J. (2019). Practicing matricentric feminist mothering. *Journal of the Motherhood Initiative for Research & Community Involvement, 10*(1/2), 83–99. Retrieved from https://jarm.journals.yorku.ca/index.php/jarm/article/view/40555

Johnson, K.A. (2021). *Call of the wild: How we heal trauma, awaken our own power, and use it for good.* Harper Wave.

Kendall-Tackett, K.A. (2010). Four research findings that will change what we think about perinatal depression. *The Journal of Perinatal Education, 19*(4), 7–9. 10.1624/105812410X530875

Polmanteer, R.S.R., Keefe, R.H., & Brownstein-Evans, C. (2019). Trauma-informed care with women diagnosed with postpartum depression: A conceptual framework. *Social Work in Health Care*, *58*(2), 220–235. 10.1080/00981389.2018.1535464

Seng, J., & Taylor, J. (Eds.). (2015). *Trauma informed care and the perinatal period*. Dunedin Academic Press Limited.

Stevens, N.R., Miller, M.L., Puetz, A.K., Padin, A.C., & Adams, N. (2021). Psychological intervention and treatment for post-traumatic stress disorder during pregnancy: A systematic review and call to action. *Journal of Traumatic Stress*, *34*, 575–585. 10.1002/jts.22641

Appendices

Appendix A: Trauma-Informed Intake Questionnaire for New Mothers/Parents

The following questions address things that are important for understanding your unique situation as a new mother or parent. They address areas that can be factors in Perinatal Mood and Anxiety Disorders (PMADs). PMADs always have several factors that must be looked at in combination. For all of these questions, feel free to indicate your answer briefly and not go into a lot of detail, if that will be stressful at this point. You can add as many details as you want, but please know you can omit answering any question if you need to. From a trauma-informed perspective, it is important to avoid unnecessary overwhelm from filling out paperwork.

Did you receive fertility treatment for this pregnancy? Have you received fertility treatment for other pregnancies? If yes, please briefly describe the type of treatment.

How many times have you been pregnant in your life, including this pregnancy?

Have you experienced miscarriages or pregnancy losses? If yes, how many and when?

If you have experienced a miscarriage or a pregnancy loss in the past, have you received support and/or grief counseling specifically for that?

How would you describe the degree to which this pregnancy was planned? Fully planned, partly, not planned, etc.?

Have you had any conflict(s) with a partner or significant or close others about the timing of this pregnancy? For example, disagreements about conceiving at all or how and when to conceive or fertility treatment?

How are you feeding/planning to feed your baby? Do you feel supported in your choice by family and providers?

Are you experiencing any issues related to feeding your baby? If so, have you gotten help from a provider, for example, a lactation consultant or a feeding specialist?

If you are breastfeeding or have breastfed in the past, have you experienced unpleasant or uncomfortable reactions, such as sadness, depressed mood, anxiety, irritability, or restlessness that occur just before milk release and continuing not more than a few minutes? If so, did you ever talk with a professional about it?

If you have breastfed in the past (for any amount of time), did you experience any change in mood or anxiety levels when you stopped producing milk? If so, please describe.

What setting did you give birth in or are you planning to give birth in? Hospital, birth center, home, etc. Do/did you have a doula or other support person?

Have you experienced any form of discrimination or disrespectful treatment from medical providers or other professionals during your prenatal, delivery, or postpartum care?

When you gave birth, did you experience things that you would describe as either traumatic or emotionally overwhelming? Please don't go into details here to prevent overwhelm; just indicate yes/no/possibly/other

Have you experienced any medical issues or complications in relation to your pregnancy, delivery, or postpartum recovery? If so, what were they? Feel free to indicate it briefly here without going into details.

Do you have any autoimmune illnesses? If yes, are your receiving treatment for them?

If you have been pregnant before this pregnancy, did you experience any changes in mood or anxiety during and/or after the pregnancy ended? Do you have any history of depression or anxiety or other mental health issues in relation to any previous pregnancy or fertility treatments?

If you have experienced depression, anxiety, or any other mental health issues related to fertility, pregnancy, or postpartum, did you ever receive specialized care, meaning support, care, or help from a professional specializing in working with perinatal mental health?

If you are seeing a prescriber (psychiatrist, nurse practitioner, primary care physician, OB, etc.), do you know if that person has specialized training in treating Perinatal Mood and Anxiety Disorders?

Has anyone in your family suffered from depression, anxiety, or other mental health issues in relation to pregnancy and postpartum?

Has anyone not related but close to you suffered from depression, anxiety, or other mental health issues in relation to pregnancy and postpartum? If yes, how did that impact you?

Have you gotten your thyroid and hormones checked at any point in relation to this pregnancy or postpartum period? If yes, what were the results? If not, have you discussed with any medical provider getting it checked?

How do you feel about the level of support you have from family and friends?

Do you have a history of either a formal diagnosis or any symptoms of Premenstrual Dysphoric Disorder? Or other issues related to hormonal systems? Premenstrual Dysphoric Disorder symptoms include severe mood swings, irritability, anxiety, tension, lack of energy, changes in appetite, and changes in sleep.

How would you describe your sleep situation? Are you getting enough sleep to feel you can function, less than optimal, or are you severely sleep deprived? If you had childcare help and a quiet space for yourself, would you be able to sleep when tired?

How would you describe your relationship with your baby's pediatrician? Do you feel you can get adequate information about your child's health and development?

Are you experiencing any acute or chronic pain issues? If yes, are you receiving treatment for it?

How can a provider make you feel safe and comfortable when receiving care? What are things that help you feel safe?

Is there anything else you would like to add?

Appendix B: Somatic Self-Regulation Skills and Exercises

Skills	Exercise
Sensory awareness and differentiation	Locate the most stable or least tense part of your body. What happens when you focus on that part for a moment? Notice the difference between this sensation and other parts. You can bring your awareness back and forth between them. What do you notice when you do that?
External awareness	Notice your immediate surroundings with your senses: ♦ Let your eyes wander around the room and notice shapes, colors, light, shadows. If you have a view, see how far you can see. ♦ Listen to all sounds and notice the difference between those close by and far away. ♦ Notice any smells or textural qualities of the air. ♦ Notice the textures of items around you by touching and looking.
Grounding	Notice any sensations related to gravity: Your weight sitting on your chair, your hands resting on your legs, your back leaning against something, any contact you a making with the floor. Try to deepen the sense of gravity pulling at your body.
Checking of activation levels	Notice your pulse and heartbeat, is it faster or slower than usual? Notice the pace of your breath, the warmth in your limbs, your energy levels. On the spectrum of being at the cusp of falling asleep on one end to maximal physical exertion on the other end, where are you right now? Do you have any muscle tension or alertness, feeling ready to move?
Up- and down-regulating	Bring you awareness to either your inner sensations or your surroundings and stay there for a moment. Do you notice any changes? Do your energy levels increase or decrease? Focus on an internal sensation for a moment. Does it intensify or subside? Focus on exploring your surroundings. Notice how that changes your inner state.
Monitoring	As you bring your awareness back and forth between your inner state and your surroundings, track how your state is shifting, like waves. Observe how bringing your awareness inwards makes changes to your state that are different from when you bring your awareness outside yourself. Notice if you are continuing to build a certain state from shifting your attention around. For example, as you are exploring internal sensations of different parts of your body, notice how your sense of stability and grounding might deepen.
Regulating movements	Notice any impulses to move. Before you follow the impulse, feel into the sensations of the impulse: How the leg that is wanting to move feels like just before you move it. Then move your leg and pause to notice what it felt like. How did it change your state to

(Cont.)

Skills	Exercise
	follow the impulse? Explore any urges to make posture adjustments, including making connections between body parts, for example putting your hands on your legs. Pause and notice how the movements and self-touch affected your state. As you are exploring this, notice the experience of being in charge of how you are moving.
Slowing down	*Imagine you have pushed a button to slow down the speed of everything to slow-motion. What comes up when everything is paused? If it feels frustrating, notice this frustration without judging it. Track the urges to move that comes with it. Notice what sensations stand out in your awareness when you are slowed down. Even if you find yourself rushing to move, notice what it feels like to slow down your pace a little bit.*
Somatic agency	*As you are getting more familiar with your sensations, notice what feels effective for making you feel stable. Explore what it feels like to be in charge of how you are moving around and where you are shifting your attention. If it feels hard to change your posture or make any movements, imagine yourself making a movement that you know is related to feeling stable. What does it feel like to imagine this? Do you notice any impulses or urges to move?*
Establish relative safety	*From exploration of your inner state and your surroundings, take a moment to assess your safety right in this moment. How do you know you are relatively safe right now? What are sensations in your body that are telling you that you are relatively safe? If you are struggling to feel any safety, notice the part of your body or something in the surroundings that feels the least threatening. What sensation or object feel the safest to focus on? It can be an internal sensation or something in your immediate surroundings. When you have identified this, keep your awareness with it and deepen the experience of safety.*

Index

Page numbers in *italics* indicate figures; page numbers in **bold** indicate tables

affect regulation 5, 21, 115–116, 119, 149, 208; and treatment of PTSD 121, 152
affect tolerance 72, 119, 168, 180, 204, 206, *207*, 208
allostatic load 22–23, 85, 123, 127, 140, 185, 230, 233; *see also* toxic stress
anti-inflammatory interventions 6, **46**, 86–87, 126, 141; referral considerations 233, *234*
attachment history 4; and trauma 117, 155, 165, 185, 203, 213
attunement **46**, 75, 116–118, 120, *146*; and psychoeducation 230; and the therapeutic relationship 128–129, 131, 147–149, and trauma 117; *see also* resonance

Benjamin, J. 10, 61, 63–64, 65, 97–98, 100
biopsychosocial perspective 3–4, 7, 125–126, 140; and clinical creativity 224–226; and trauma 20, 116
body identity 74, 104, 106–107, 109–110; maternal 107–108, 111, 139, 142, *143*; shifts in maternal transition 144, 182, 228–229
body narrative 74, 106–107, 195; maternal 111, 142, *143*, 169, 182, 183, 191–193; and trauma healing 203, 205, 213, 228–229
bodyfulness 106–107, 111, 203; and empowered mothering 108, 205; *see also* maternal bodyfulness
bodylessness 6, 69–70, 104, 214; and sensory awareness 106–107, 186; *see also* maternal bodylessness

bottom-up interventions 115–117, 120; and somatic psychotherapy 118, 177

Caldwell, C.M. 6, 14, 69, 74, 104, 106–110, 131, 139, 144, 157, 158, 169, 178, 182, 183, 186, 191
childhood maltreatment/abuse 26–27, 37, 152, 204; and perinatal PTSD 40, 124–125; and sensory awareness 185; and trauma healing 213–214
clinical creativity 224–226
clinical skills 144–146, 151; attunement and resonance 155–156; *see also* nervous system tracking; sensory awareness skills
clinician self-reflection 172; questions 172–173
coregulation 5, 9, 11, 35, **46**; and nervous system tracking 180–181; in the perinatal period 147–149, 177; and repair 151; research findings 87, 117, 141; and resonance 151; and telehealth 171; and the therapeutic relationship 116–118, 120, 129–131, 144, 143, 157; and trauma 127, 152–154
countertransference *see* somatic countertransference

discrimination 30, 44, 68, 85, 104, 125, 142; and intersectional perspective 100; trauma-informed intake question 240
dissociation 39–41, 68, 70, 155, 185, 196, 210
dysregulation: and bodylessness 105; different from somatic countertransference 167; endocrinological 81–82; nervous

system 42, 72–73, 87, 119, 185; perinatal specific 144, 148–149, 160–162; and PMADs 160; and resonance 160–161, 169; and trauma 152, 159, 179, 196; treatment of 120, 127, 144, 158

embodied relational subjectivity 71–73, 75, 192
emotion regulation 176–177; and sensory awareness 177–178; *see also* affect tolerance
empowered mothering 7, 15, 93, 101–103; different from feminist mothering 102; five tenets of 103; and maternal bodyfulness 108–110, 184; and trauma-informed care 111; in treatment strategy 139, *140*, 142, 205, 229
exteroception 158, 159, 177, 181, **209**

feminist mothering 93–94, 101, 108–109, 142; different from empowered mothering 102; and trauma-informed care 111
feminist psychoanalysis 4–5, 9–10, 60–63; informing clinical work 71–74; integrative model 139, *140*; and maternal subjectivity 66–67; and matricentric feminism 97–98

health inequity 30–31, 44, 85, 145

iatrogenic effects of obstetric care 19, 27–28, 84, 124
inflammation 22; and depression 79–82; and pain 41; and PTSD/trauma 27, 126; and social support 87
institutionalized motherhood 12, 63, 66–67, 92, 100, 102; dictates of 96; and sensory awareness 181
intensive mothering 7, 94–97, 110; and Maternal Mental Health 98–99, 141; and maternal sense of self 183–184; psychological functions of 100; and racial discrimination 30; resisting 196; *see also* patriarchal motherhood
interoception 158, 159, 176–177, 180–181; and nervous system tracking 119, 157–158, 189, **209**, 213; *see also* sensory awareness
intimate partner violence 32, 36

Levine, P.A. 14, 20, 22, 26, 34, 83, 88, 116, 119, 120, 125, 126, 130, 131, 139, 148, 150, 157, 158, 159, 178, 179, 182, 184, 187, 195, 206, 207, 208

maternal bodyfulness 6, 106–107, 139, 193, 195–196; and sensory awareness 183; as empowered mothering 108–109; as treatment strategy 142, 143; and somatic countertransference 168; and trauma healing 204–206, *207*, 214, 226; cycle of empowerment 227
maternal bodylessness 104–106, 108, 129, 140, *141*, 145; and intensive mothering 164; and shame 155; and somatic receptivity 163
maternal brain plasticity 79–80, 85, 126, 177; and healing 88, 141
maternal identity formation/development 60–61, 74, 128; and sensory awareness 182–183; and trauma healing 205; *see also* maternal sense of self; maternal subjectivity
Maternal Mental Health 6: definition of field 10; developments in 7–8, 13; disparities in 4, 6, 11, 44, 47, 31, 100, 125, 142; screening 7, 24, 41, 43, 83
maternal sense of self 103, 107, 148, 177; and intensive mothering 183–184; and sensory awareness and pleasure 179, 182–184, 188; and trauma 130–131, 155, 185; *see also* maternal subjectivity
maternal subjectivity 4–5, 10, 97, 132; and bodylessness 104, 108; denial/erasure of 64, 129, 140, 191; and embodiment

64, 67, 71–72, 100, 102, 148, 168–169; and sensory awareness 178, 183; as theoretical problem 61–63, 64; and trauma 69–71, 130–131, 185; and trauma healing 204–205, 214
maternal trauma healing 109, 200–205; cyclical nature of 202, 228; and timing of trauma treatment
matricentric feminism 5–7, 63, 92–94; intersectional approach 100, 125; as lived praxis 101–102; overview of 97–98; and perinatal trauma healing 109, 111, *140*, 205, 225; understanding of bodylessness 105

nervous system: regulation 116, 126, *140*, 211; tracking 139, 144, *146*, 151, 155–158; tracking as clinical skill 157–159; tracking for self-regulation 189–190; tracking and psychoeducation 166

O'Reilly, A. 6, 62, 63, 92–97, 99–103, 109–111, 139
Obsessive Compulsive Disorder 38–39
Orbach, S. 15, 61, 65–66, 69, 72–74, 132, 150, 155, 160, 165, 167, 168, 169, 186, 187, 206
oxytocin 79–81, 86, 123

pandemic stress 7, 32; and telehealth 170
patriarchal motherhood 7, 67, 70, 93–94, 96–97, 102–103, 125; and bodylessness 104–105, 108, 110, 129, 164; resisting 184, 196, 205; as target of treatment 139, 141; *see also* intensive mothering
Perinatal Mood and Anxiety Disorders (PMADs) 3, 8, 24, 99, 126, 128; anxiety 123, 128; biomarkers 123; comorbidity with trauma 23, 82; and dysregulation 160; and inflammation 82; interactions with trauma 86, 128; prevalence 7, 23; reproductive biology 81, 84, 85; *see also* postpartum anxiety; postpartum depression

perinatal trauma 127; and comorbidity 23, 41; definition 19, 35; types of 26; *see also* trauma
perinatal/maternal somatic themes 144, 148, 154, 156, 172, 196
polyvagal theory 122
Porges, S.W. 22, 34–35, 120, 122, 147, 153, 164
post-traumatic stress disorder (PTSD) 19, 119; clinical vignette 214; and comorbidity with PMADs 21–23, 41; diagnostic criteria 21; general prevalence 21; partial 22; perinatal specific 23–24, 28–29, 35, 38, 42, 124; prevalence in perinatal period 8, 23–25; as risk factor for PMADs 24, 27, 123; *see also* trauma
post-traumatic stress symptoms 35, 41; *see also* trauma symptoms
postpartum anxiety 123, 128
postpartum depression 3, 6–7, 28, 30–32, 37, 41, 43–45, 61, 68; and anger 43; and inflammation 3, 79–82; and intensive mothering ideology 99; research on 128, 170; and sexual abuse history 31; and sleep disturbances 36, 82; and traumatic childbirth 28
pregnancy and infant loss 5, 29–30, 238; treatment of 211–213
preterm delivery 27–28, 30, 125
proprioception 119, 158, 159, 177, 180, **209**
psychoeducation **46**, 153, 200, 202, 227, 227; and dysregulation 166; and nervous system tracking 158–159; on perinatal trauma 229–230, **231-232**; and sensory awareness 181, 189; and sensory vocabulary 193, **194**; and somatic receptivity 164; and telehealth 171
psychoneuroimmunology 3, 82, 85, 141

relational safety 118, 126; and the therapeutic relationship 120, 153 resonance 75, 118, *146*, 150–151, 156–157, 205; and psychoeducation 230; and repair 151; and telehealth 171

Schore, A.N. 8–10, 26, 35, 115–121, 128, 144, 147, 150, 151, 154, 157, 183
self-regulation: changes in maternal transition 124, 182; and developmental history 182; skills and exercises 161–162, 189–190, **191**, 243–244; in somatic psychotherapy 120, 126, 129–130, 179, 186, 189; and telehealth 171; and therapeutic relationship 187; and trauma 152, 184–186
Selvam, R. 150–151, 155, 157, 161, 162, 167–168, 171, 180, 208, 213
sensory awareness 132, 142, *143*, 145; and agency 179; and coregulation 158; and developmental history 157; and experiential capacity 184, 204–206; and flashbacks 208, **209**; foundations of 180–182; introducing skills to perinatal clients 180, 188–198, 243; reflection questions 188; and resonance 150; and sexual abuse history 32; skills 37, 130, *146*, 189–190; and trauma treatment 119, 184, 186–187
sensory vocabulary 110, 131, 142, *143*, *146*, 188, 191–193; psychoeducation on 193, **194**
sexual abuse 26, 31–32, 124, 184
shame 41, 99, **106**, 165, 193; clinical vignette 217; and clinician self-reflection 172; and coregulation 154–155
slowing down 159, 178, *182*, 196, 203, 244; clinical vignette 221
somatic agency 179–181, *182*, 189, 191, 196, 201, 244
somatic countertransference 72, 139, *140*, 143–145, 167–169, 187; and maternal themes 172; *see also* clinician self-reflection

Somatic Experiencing 2, 119–121; *see also* Levine, P.A.
somatic psychotherapy: integrated with psychoanalysis 74, 116, 128, 130–132, 139; integrative model *140*; rationale for use in perinatal period 127–130; scientific background for 118–121
somatic receptivity 72, 145, *146*, 163–164, 184, 213; and psychoeducation 164; and somatic countertransference 168; and trauma 164–167
stillbirth 29–30; *see also* pregnancy and infant loss

telehealth 170–172; and resonance 171
therapeutic relationship *see* attunement; resonance; somatic countertransference; therapeutic safety
therapeutic safety 42, 122, 144–145, *146*, 189, 192, 200–201
toxic stress 22–23, 126, 185, 230, 233; *see also* allostatic load
trauma: attachment 1, 80–81, 88, 213; betrayal 44, 125; definition of 19–20; delayed onset 35; impact on coregulation 127, 152–154; impact on self-regulation 152, 184–186; impact on sensory awareness 70, 184–185; impact on therapeutic relationship 161; and psychoeducation 227; risks and vulnerability in the perinatal period 11, 82, 125; treatment and telehealth 171; *see also* trauma symptoms
trauma-informed care: intake questionnaire 238–242; and matricentric feminism 111; principles of 45–47, 126–127, 170–171, 224, 229
trauma-sensitive treatment planning 152, 202, 224–226
trauma symptoms: anger, rage, and irritability 34, 43–44, 125, 185; avoidance and

dissociation 39–41, 155, 185, 196, 210; delayed onset 35, 202; flashbacks and intrusive thoughts 38–39, 208; hyperarousal and reactivity/hypervigilance 42–43, 125, 153, 164, 193; negative mood or cognitions 21, 41–42; in the perinatal period 8, 33–36, 40, 68; sleep disturbances 36–38; suicidality 39, 44; and traumatic childbirth 28–29; traumatized body self 40, 61, 68–70; *see also* dissociation; post-traumatic stress disorder; traumatic memories

traumatic childbirth 5, 24, 26–29, 33, 38–39, 43–44, 83, 184; clinical vignette 214; definition of 29; and healing process 203, 208, 210–211; risk factors 84; and sensory vocabulary 192; and sexual abuse history 31; trauma-informed intake question 240

traumatic memories 24, 32, 38–39, 120, 129, 142, 159, 185, 193, 195; processing of *207*–208, 212; protocol for processing flashbacks **209**; *see also* dissociation

traumatic stress 22, 127, 140, 179, 185, 204; and birth outcome disparities 31, 125; after childbirth 25; and flashbacks 208

treatment goals and strategy 142–143, 227–229, 234, **235**; and telehealth 171

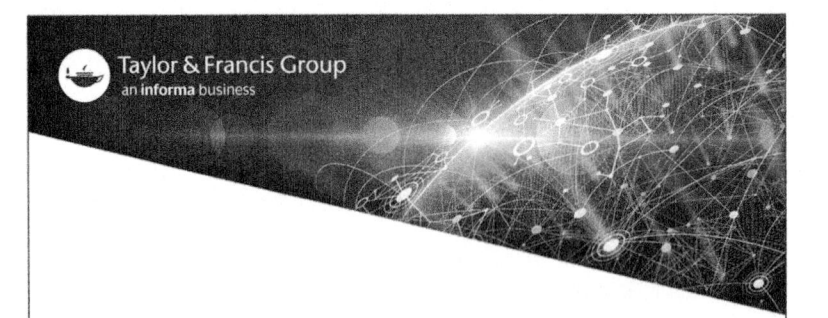

Printed in Great Britain
by Amazon